*"The Psychological Depth of Disease and Homoeopathy"*

# The Soul of Sickness

By Dr. Vikrant R Mishra
MD(Hom)

*Founder,*
***Horizon Multispeciality Homoeopathy***
*Assistant Professor,*
***Smt. V.N. Vyas Homoeopathic Medical College***
*Former Lecturer,*
***Practice of Medicine, Shri B.A. Dangar Homoeopathic Medical College***

A Homoeopathic Exploration of Psychodynamics

**The Soul of Sickness**

*The Psychological Depth of Disease and Homoeopathy"*

ISBN: 978-93-342-6922-2

Published by Dr.Vikrant Rajnath Mishra



For permissions, contact:
Email: Vikrant_mishra2003@yahoo.com

# Table of Contents

# Preface

For centuries, healers and philosophers have recognized that **disease is not merely a physical affliction but an emotional and spiritual crisis**. Yet, modern medicine often treats symptoms in isolation, overlooking the deeper causes that shape illness. homoeopathy, however, embraces a different perspective—one that sees disease as a meaningful dialogue between the psyche and the body.

Throughout my practice, I have witnessed countless cases where chronic conditions were directly linked to **emotional suppression, childhood trauma, grief, or deep-seated fears**. Patients struggling with migraines carried unresolved anger. Individuals with autoimmune diseases often bore the emotional burden of guilt and self-punishment. Skin disorders revealed long-standing grief, while hormonal imbalances pointed to suppressed identity conflicts.

These are not coincidences. They are **expressions of the soul's distress, encoded in the body's language**.

This book is an **invitation to rethink disease**—not as a battle to be fought, but as a lesson to be understood. By combining **Homoeopathic case-taking with psychological insights**, we can uncover the true nature of illness and guide patients toward lasting transformation.

For practitioners, this book offers **a structured approach to understanding the emotional depth behind physical ailments**. For patients, it provides a **path to self-awareness**

**and healing**, helping them recognize the hidden messages behind their symptoms.

Healing is not just about curing; it is about **understanding the soul's journey through sickness and health**. May this book serve as a guide to **decoding the mind-body connection and unlocking the true essence of holistic healing**.

**Dr. Vikrant R. Mishra**
*MD(Hom)*

## Introduction

*Health is not merely the absence of disease; it is a delicate balance between the body, mind, and soul. Yet, when this balance is disturbed, illness emerges—not as an arbitrary affliction but as a profound communication from the subconscious. Disease, in its essence, is the body's way of narrating a deeper, unspoken story.*

This book, *The Soul of Sickness*, delves into the **psychological depth of disease**, exploring how suppressed emotions, unresolved traumas, and hidden conflicts manifest as physical symptoms. In homoeopathy, we recognize that every symptom holds meaning, every ailment carries a message, and every cure lies in understanding this intricate interplay between mind and body.

By integrating **psychodynamic principles with Homoeopathic wisdom**, this book seeks to uncover the unseen forces shaping disease, guiding practitioners and patients toward true healing.

### Why This Book?

In conventional medicine, disease is often seen as a mechanical dysfunction—organs failing, cells misbehaving, and biochemical processes going awry. However, homoeopathy teaches us that disease is far more than just physical pathology; it is **an expression of inner disharmony**. This book explores:

- **The symbolism of disease**—how physical symptoms reveal psychological struggles.

- **The emotional roots of chronic illness**—how stress, fear, and suppression create disease patterns.
- **homoeopathy as a psychodynamic tool**—how remedies help resolve both emotional conflicts and physical suffering.
- **The vital force and energy medicine**—how the unseen life force influences health and illness.
- **Real-life case studies**—demonstrating the mind-body connection in Homoeopathic healing.

By understanding the **language of disease**, we can **transform suffering into self-awareness and healing**.

**Dr.Vikrant R Mishra**

**MD(Hom)**

## Acknowledgment

This book is a product of immense learning and support from many wonderful people, to whom I am deeply grateful.

**My Patients – My Greatest Teachers**

Your trust and experiences have shaped my understanding of homoeopathy and continue to inspire my practice.

**A Tribute to My Father**

I dedicate this book to my father, *Swargiya Rajnath Mishra*, whose values and blessings guide me every day.

**Gratitude to My Guru**

A special thanks to *Dr. Milind Rao Sir*, whose wisdom and mentorship have profoundly influenced my journey in homoeopathy.

**Unwavering Support from Teachers & Friends**

I sincerely appreciate *Dr. Jitendra Mishra* for his encouragement, *Chandraprakash Yadav* and *Jagdish Nishad* for their constant support, and *Dr. M. Hulikatti, Dr. Pratap, Dr. Ramakant, Dr. Madhuri, Dr. Ashis, Jwala, Vaibhav, Pritam, Hemant, and Bharat* for always being there.

**My Pillars of Strength**

My deepest gratitude to my mother, *Rekha Mishra*, and my wife, *Dr. Bilkis (Dr. Poonam Mishra)*, for their unwavering love, support, and belief in my work.

To all of you—this book is a reflection of your encouragement and faith. Thank you!

**Dr. Vikrant R. Mishra**
*MD (Hom)*

## Chapter (0):Shoonya: The Silent Origin

> *"In the beginning, there was no symptom, no suffering, no separation—only stillness. That stillness is Shoonya."*

Shoonya is not emptiness in the hollow sense—it is **full potential**. It is the unmanifest, the eternal canvas from which all life arises.

We are not merely bodies with symptoms.
We are **beings composed of three interwoven realities**:

- **Soul** – the eternal observer, formless and unborn
- **Mind** – the field of emotions, thoughts, and responses
- **Body** – the visible expression, the stage where the story unfolds

---

### The Descent into Disease

Disease does not begin in the body.
It begins in the **disruption of soul-consciousness** — a misalignment with our deeper truth.

- When the **soul** forgets its nature or is overshadowed by trauma, isolation, or suppression of being,
- The **mind** starts to distort: emotions become exaggerated, thoughts become reactive, identity becomes fragmented.
- Eventually, the **body** bears the burden — expressing the soul's silent scream through symptoms and syndromes.

What we call "illness" is often the **final echo** of an internal disharmony that started much earlier.

> *"The body speaks when the soul has been silenced."*

---

**Why Begin with Shoonya?**

This book begins with **Shoonya** because healing must begin with **remembrance** — the remembering of who we are beneath the noise of suffering.

Shoonya is the **baseline**—not of nothingness, but of wholeness.
Before the first symptom… there was balance.
Before imbalance… there was soul-awareness.

In this still space of Shoonya, healing begins.

---

**The Pattern of Manifestation**

- From **Soul**, disturbance arises
- It descends into the **Mind**, altering perceptions, beliefs, emotions
- Finally, it takes shape in the **Body**, where it becomes visible

This is the sacred **downward spiral of disease**. And healing is simply the **upward return** — from physical relief, to emotional resolution, to **soul realignment**.

> *"True healing does not end with the disappearance of symptoms.*
> *It ends with the return to Shoonya — to the stillness from which health was first born."*

---

# Chapter 1: Understanding the Mind and Its Influence on the Body

### Introduction

The mind is the command center of human existence, governing thoughts, emotions, and behaviour. It is divided into the conscious and subconscious realms, both of which play a crucial role in overall health. While the conscious mind is responsible for logical thinking and decision-making, the subconscious stores deep-seated emotions, memories, and patterns that influence physical health in ways we may not always recognize.

---

### The Physiological Effects of Emotions

Emotions are not just psychological states; they have profound physiological effects. The body reacts to different emotions through chemical and neurological responses, altering heart rate, blood pressure, hormone levels, and immune function. This interplay between mind and body forms the basis of psychosomatic health.

For example:

- **Anger:** When a person becomes angry, the body enters a heightened state of arousal. The adrenal glands release **adrenaline and cortisol**, leading to increased heart rate, elevated blood pressure, and faster breathing. Blood is redirected to the muscles in preparation for a fight-or-flight response. Physiological signs include a flushed face, tightened muscles, and sometimes palpitations.
- **Fear and Anxiety:** In response to fear or anxiety, the body activates the **sympathetic nervous system**, triggering the release of **noradrenaline**. This causes blood vessels to constrict, leading to cold hands and feet. The heart may

race, breathing becomes shallow, and digestion slows down as the body prioritizes survival over non-essential functions.

- **Happiness and Relaxation:** Positive emotions trigger the release of **dopamine, serotonin, and oxytocin**, which promote relaxation, lower stress hormone levels, and enhance overall well-being. The parasympathetic nervous system activates, leading to lower heart rate, improved digestion, and a sense of calm.

### Types of Emotions and Their Physiological Impact

Emotions can be broadly categorized into:

- **Primary Emotions** (innate, universal responses such as joy, sadness, fear, anger, surprise, and disgust)
- **Secondary Emotions** (shaped by personal experiences and cultural influences, such as shame, guilt, pride, and jealousy)

Each of these emotions carries unique physiological imprints that, when prolonged or suppressed, can contribute to disease development. For example:

- **Chronic stress and fear** can lead to high cortisol levels, increasing the risk of hypertension, digestive disorders, and immune suppression.
- **Suppressed anger** may contribute to liver dysfunction and hypertension.
- **Unresolved grief** can manifest as respiratory disorders like asthma.

Understanding these links allows us to see how psychological states influence physical health.

---

# Chapter 2: Understanding the Mind

## What is the Mind?

The **mind** is the seat of consciousness, thought, emotions, and perception. It is an intangible yet powerful entity that governs our awareness, decision-making, memory, and behaviour. While the brain is the physical organ that processes information, the mind is the **non-material aspect** that interprets, analyzes, and responds to experiences. It shapes our reality and plays a crucial role in our health and well-being.

The mind is often classified into different layers based on its depth of awareness and function. Various philosophical, psychological, and neuroscientific models attempt to explain the workings of the mind, but all agree that it is a **dynamic, ever-evolving system** that influences every aspect of human existence.

---

## Layers of the Mind

The mind is commonly divided into three levels, each with distinct characteristics:

| Layer of the Mind | Description | Functions | Influence on Behaviour |
|---|---|---|---|
| **Conscious Mind** | The part we are actively aware of in daily life. | Logical thinking, decision-making, short-term memory. | Governs rational thought and voluntary actions. |
| **Subconscious Mind** | A hidden layer that stores emotions, habits, and learned | Controls automatic responses, deep-seated beliefs, and emotional conditioning. | Shapes personality, reactions, and instincts. |

| | behaviours. | | |
|---|---|---|---|
| **Unconscious Mind** | The deepest layer, housing instincts, suppressed memories, and inherited patterns. | Manages primitive drives, repressed experiences, and trauma. | Can manifest in subconscious fears, dreams, or psychosomatic illnesses. |

*Each layer of the mind plays a crucial role in shaping our reality, health, and responses to life experiences. The subconscious and unconscious levels often drive our behaviours without us being fully aware of them.*

---

**Functions of the Mind**

The mind performs various functions essential for survival, emotional well-being, and self-development:

1. **Perception and Awareness**
    - The mind processes sensory information and constructs reality based on past experiences and beliefs.
    - It interprets external stimuli such as sight, sound, taste, touch, and smell, assigning meaning to them.
2. **Thinking and Decision-Making**
    - The conscious mind engages in reasoning, problem-solving, and analysis.
    - The subconscious mind influences decisions based on habits, emotions, and past experiences.
3. **Memory and Learning**

- The mind stores information in short-term, long-term, and procedural memory.
- It retrieves past experiences to guide current actions and behaviours.

4. **Emotional Regulation**
    - The mind manages emotional responses to situations.
    - It controls fear, joy, anger, sadness, and other emotions through biochemical and neural processes.

5. **Imagination and Creativity**
    - The subconscious mind plays a crucial role in creative thinking and problem-solving.
    - Dreams and intuition arise from deeper layers of the mind.

6. **Autonomic and Habitual Functions**
    - The subconscious mind regulates involuntary bodily functions like breathing, digestion, and heart rate.
    - It also manages learned habits and reflexive responses.

---

### The Relationship Between the Mind and the Brain

While the **brain** is the physical structure made up of neurons, the **mind** is the non-physical entity that interprets, thinks, and feels. The two are deeply interconnected, as the brain provides the biological foundation for mental processes. Neuroscientists often describe the brain as the "hardware" and the mind as the "software" running on it.

Key aspects of their relationship:

- The **brain** processes sensory inputs, while the **mind** interprets them.
- The **brain** releases neurotransmitters (such as serotonin, dopamine, and adrenaline), affecting emotions and mental states.
- Mental states such as stress, joy, and anxiety influence brain chemistry and bodily health.

---

**The Mind as an Energy System**

The mind can also be understood as an **energy field** that interacts with the body. Psychological theories suggest that thoughts and emotions carry vibrational frequencies that affect overall well-being. This concept aligns with holistic healing approaches, including homoeopathy, where mental and emotional imbalances contribute to disease.

According to this view:

- Positive thoughts generate **harmonious energy**, promoting health.
- Negative emotions create **disharmony**, potentially leading to physical illness.

---

### Conclusion

*The mind is a vast and complex entity that influences every aspect of human life. It is responsible for perception, thought, memory, emotions, and subconscious conditioning. Understanding the layers and functions of the mind helps in recognizing how emotional and psychological factors shape health and disease.*

---

## Chapter 3: The Role of Emotions in Brain Development

### Introduction

The journey of brain development begins in the **womb**, where the foundation of neurological growth is laid. During this period, a baby is deeply influenced by the mother's emotional and physical state. Scientific research and holistic health systems, including homoeopathy, emphasize that the mother's emotions have a profound impact on the developing child, shaping not only brain function but also future emotional patterns and personality traits.

This chapter explores how emotions, particularly those experienced by the mother, influence brain development from the earliest stages of life.

---

### 1. Brain Development in the Womb: The Emotional Connection

The fetus begins its neurological development early in pregnancy. By the **third week of gestation**, the neural tube forms, which later develops into the **brain and spinal cord**. During this phase, various factors influence the baby's brain, but one of the most significant is the **emotional state of the mother**.

The **maternal emotional environment** plays a key role in brain wiring. Emotional experiences of the mother—whether positive or negative—result in the release of biochemical signals that **cross the placenta** and shape fetal brain structure. These biochemical signals include stress hormones, neurotransmitters, and other neuropeptides, which influence:

- Neuronal growth
- Brain plasticity
- Cognitive functions
- Emotional resilience or vulnerability

---

## 2. How Maternal Emotions Affect Fetal Brain Development

### A. Stress and Fear

When a mother experiences **chronic stress, anxiety, or fear**, high levels of **cortisol** (the stress hormone) circulate in her bloodstream. These hormones cross the placenta and enter the developing fetus, affecting:

- The **amygdala**, the brain's fear-processing centre, which may become **hyperactive**, leading to a heightened stress response in the child.
- The **hippocampus**, which regulates memory and learning, potentially affecting cognitive abilities.
- The **prefrontal cortex**, which governs rational thinking and decision-making, leading to increased risk of emotional instability.

◈ **Example:** Studies show that babies exposed to high maternal stress levels in utero are more likely to develop **anxiety disorders,**

**hyper-reactivity to stress, and emotional dysregulation** later in life.

---

### B. Love and Positive Emotions

Conversely, when a mother experiences **love, joy, and emotional stability**, her body releases **endorphins, oxytocin, and serotonin**. These hormones create a **calming, nourishing** environment for the baby's brain development, promoting:

- **Healthy neuronal connections**, which support intelligence and emotional balance.
- **Stronger stress regulation mechanisms**, allowing the child to develop resilience against future anxiety and depression.
- **Better bonding capacity**, as oxytocin enhances the ability to form secure attachments.

◈ **Example:** A mother who feels emotionally supported and nurtured during pregnancy often gives birth to a baby with a **calmer temperament and stronger emotional adaptability**.

---

## 3. The Critical Role of the Mother-Baby Bond

Beyond the womb, emotional development continues in **infancy**. The baby's early emotional experiences—especially with the mother—determine the quality of their brain's **emotional circuitry**.

Key factors influencing this development include:

- **Skin-to-skin contact** after birth, which stimulates oxytocin and enhances bonding.

- **Mother's voice and expressions**, which regulate the baby's emotional state.
- **Responsive caregiving**, which builds a secure attachment and fosters emotional intelligence.

Infants who receive **consistent love, attention, and security** develop a well-balanced **limbic system**, which is responsible for emotional processing. Conversely, emotional neglect or chronic maternal distress may lead to **hyperactive stress responses** and emotional difficulties later in life.

---

### 4. Homoeopathic Perspective on Emotional Development in Early Life

homoeopathy recognizes that emotional imprints during fetal development can influence a child's **constitutional makeup**. Remedies that address deep-seated emotional disturbances from **gestation and early childhood** include:

| Homoeopathic Remedy | Indications |
|---|---|
| **Natrum Muriaticum** | For individuals who internalize early emotional pain and grief. |
| **Aurum Metallicum** | Helps in overcoming deep-seated sadness and emotional suppression. |
| **Pulsatilla** | Beneficial for individuals who need warmth, love, and emotional reassurance. |
| **Staphysagria** | Addresses suppressed emotions, particularly those stemming from early trauma. |

---

### Conclusion

*The emotional environment during pregnancy plays a* ***vital role in shaping brain development****. A mother's stress, joy, love, or fear leaves lasting imprints on the child's brain, influencing emotional resilience, cognitive abilities, and future personality. Understanding this connection allows for better prenatal care, emotional support for mothers, and preventive interventions to ensure* ***healthy emotional development from the earliest stages of life****.*

---

## Chapter 4:Neuronal Growth, Brain Plasticity, Cognitive Functions, and Emotional Resilience

### Introduction

The human brain is a dynamic and adaptable structure, constantly evolving through experiences, emotions, and learning. At the core of this adaptability lies **neuronal growth**, **brain plasticity**, **cognitive functions**, and **emotional resilience**—four fundamental aspects that determine intellectual and emotional development.

These processes begin in the womb and continue throughout life, shaping how individuals perceive, react, and adapt to their environment. Understanding these aspects provides insight into how emotions, experiences, and even Homoeopathic interventions influence overall mental and physical well-being.

---

### 1. Neuronal Growth: Building the Brain's Foundation

Neuronal growth, or **neurogenesis**, refers to the formation of new neurons. This process is most active during fetal development but continues in certain brain regions throughout life, particularly in the **hippocampus** (responsible for memory and learning).

**Factors Influencing Neuronal Growth:**

- **Prenatal Environment:** Proper nutrition, maternal emotional stability, and the absence of toxic substances promote healthy neuronal development.
- **Postnatal Stimulation:** Sensory experiences, learning, and emotional bonding stimulate neuronal connections.
- **Exercise and Mental Activity:** Engaging in new learning activities and physical exercise enhances neurogenesis.
- **Stress and Trauma:** Chronic stress or emotional trauma can impair neuronal growth, particularly in regions linked to memory and emotional regulation.

◈ **Example:** Studies show that children who grow up in emotionally supportive environments have **denser neuronal connections**, leading to improved problem-solving and emotional adaptability.

---

### 2. Brain Plasticity: The Adaptability of the Mind

**Neuroplasticity**, or brain plasticity, is the ability of the brain to reorganize itself by forming new neural connections in response to learning, experience, and emotional stimuli. This process allows the brain to recover from injuries, adapt to new situations, and refine skills over time.

**Types of Brain Plasticity:**

| Type | Description | Example |
|---|---|---|
| **Developmental Plasticity** | Occurs naturally as the brain grows and matures. | A child learning a language effortlessly. |

| | | |
|---|---|---|
| **Adaptive Plasticity** | The brain compensates for damage or learning deficits. | A stroke patient relearning movement. |
| **Experience-Dependent Plasticity** | The brain strengthens connections based on experience and learning. | Practicing a musical instrument enhances coordination. |

**Emotions and Brain Plasticity**

- **Positive emotions** like love and happiness enhance neural connectivity and increase adaptability.
- **Chronic stress** reduces plasticity, impairing cognitive and emotional flexibility.
- **Mindfulness and meditation** boost plasticity by reducing stress hormones and enhancing memory functions.

◈ **Example:** London taxi drivers develop a larger **hippocampus** due to the extensive mental mapping required for navigation, demonstrating the impact of experience on brain structure.

---

### 3. Cognitive Functions: The Pillars of Thought and Perception

Cognitive functions refer to the **mental processes** that enable individuals to acquire knowledge, understand experiences, and make decisions. These functions are shaped by both genetic and environmental factors, including emotional experiences.

**Core Cognitive Functions:**

| Function | Role in the Mind |
|---|---|
| **Attention** | Focuses on relevant stimuli while ignoring |

| | |
|---|---|
| | distractions. |
| **Memory** | Stores and retrieves information for learning and decision-making. |
| **Problem-Solving** | Analyzes situations and develops solutions. |
| **Language Processing** | Enables communication and interpretation of meaning. |
| **Executive Functioning** | Controls planning, impulse regulation, and goal setting. |

**How Emotions Influence Cognition**

- **Positive emotions** enhance creativity, problem-solving, and memory recall.
- **Negative emotions** (like chronic fear or sadness) reduce cognitive flexibility and decision-making efficiency.
- **Trauma and stress** impair memory and executive function, often leading to cognitive decline.

◈ **Example:** Anxiety often leads to **overthinking and difficulty concentrating**, as the brain prioritizes survival responses over rational thought.

---

**4. Emotional Resilience: Strengthening the Mind Against Stress**

**Emotional resilience** is the ability to **adapt to stress, trauma, and adversity** without long-term psychological harm. It is shaped by early-life experiences, brain plasticity, and emotional regulation mechanisms.

**Key Components of Emotional Resilience:**

1. **Self-Awareness:** Understanding one's emotions and triggers.
2. **Cognitive Reframing:** Changing negative thought patterns into positive perspectives.
3. **Social Support:** Strong emotional connections help regulate stress responses.
4. **Stress Management Techniques:** Meditation, breathing exercises, and self-care strengthen resilience.
5. **Homoeopathic Support:** Remedies like *Ignatia*, *Natrum Muriaticum*, and *Aconitum* help regulate emotional responses.

◈ **Example:** People who practice mindfulness and gratitude develop a **stronger prefrontal cortex**, allowing them to handle stress more effectively.

---

**Conclusion**

*The brain is a constantly evolving organ, influenced by* ***neuronal growth, plasticity, cognitive functions, and emotional resilience****. Emotions play a crucial role in shaping these aspects, either enhancing or hindering mental and emotional well-being. Understanding these principles helps in designing* ***holistic approaches*** *to mental health, including emotional regulation strategies and Homoeopathic interventions.*

---

# Chapter 5: Emotions in Depth

## Introduction

Emotions are fundamental to human experience, shaping our thoughts, actions, and physiological responses. They are not merely psychological phenomena but deeply intertwined with brain function, neurochemistry, and overall health. Understanding emotions in depth requires an exploration of their origins, classifications, physiological effects, and their role in mental and physical well-being.

This chapter delves into the intricate world of emotions, from their biological underpinnings to their impact on disease and healing.

---

## 1. What Are Emotions?

Emotions are complex **psychophysiological responses** triggered by stimuli that are processed by the brain. They involve a combination of:

- **Neurological responses** (activation of brain regions like the amygdala, hypothalamus, and prefrontal cortex).
- **Hormonal changes** (release of neurotransmitters such as dopamine, serotonin, oxytocin, and cortisol).
- **Physiological effects** (changes in heart rate, respiration, blood pressure, and muscle tension).
- **Subjective experiences** (the feeling aspect of emotions, such as joy, sadness, or anger).
- **Behavioral expressions** (facial expressions, body language, and vocal tone).

◈ **Example:** When a person encounters a threatening situation, the brain quickly processes the information and triggers a **fear response**, leading to increased heartbeat, sweating, and heightened alertness.

---

## 2. The Neuroscience of Emotions

Emotions are regulated by various brain structures that work together to process experiences and generate appropriate responses. The key components involved in emotional regulation are:

| Brain Structure | Function in Emotions |
|---|---|
| **Amygdala** | Processes fear, anger, and survival instincts. |
| **Prefrontal Cortex** | Controls emotional responses, rational thinking, and decision-making. |
| **Hippocampus** | Stores emotional memories, influencing future reactions. |
| **Hypothalamus** | Regulates autonomic responses like sweating, heartbeat, and hormone release. |
| **Anterior Cingulate Cortex** | Helps in empathy, impulse control, and emotional pain regulation. |

◈ **Example:** In patients with damage to the prefrontal cortex, emotional regulation becomes difficult, leading to impulsive behaviors and mood swings.

---

## 3. Classification of Emotions

Emotions can be broadly categorized into **primary** and **secondary** emotions:

**A. Primary Emotions** (Innate and Universal)

These are fundamental emotions present in all humans, often recognized across different cultures:

1. **Happiness** – Associated with dopamine and serotonin release.
2. **Sadness** – Often linked to lower serotonin and increased stress hormones.
3. **Fear** – Triggers the fight-or-flight response via the amygdala.
4. **Anger** – Involves heightened adrenaline and noradrenaline release.
5. **Disgust** – A survival-based reaction to avoid harmful substances.
6. **Surprise** – Prepares the brain to process unexpected events quickly.

**B. Secondary Emotions** (Developed through Experience and Social Conditioning)

These emotions arise from combinations of primary emotions and social influences:

- **Guilt** (combination of fear and sadness)
- **Shame** (linked to self-perception and social norms)
- **Love** (a mix of happiness, trust, and attachment)
- **Jealousy** (a blend of anger, insecurity, and fear)
- **Pride** (positive reinforcement of achievements)

◈ **Example:** Love is a secondary emotion that combines **attachment (oxytocin release)** with **pleasure (dopamine activation)**.

---

### 4. The Physiology of Emotions

Emotions trigger specific physiological responses that prepare the body for action. These changes include:

| Emotion | Physiological Effect |
|---|---|
| **Fear & Anxiety** | Increased heart rate, dilated pupils, cold extremities (due to blood redirection to major muscles). |
| **Anger** | Increased adrenaline, blood pressure surge, muscle tension. |
| **Sadness** | Reduced energy, slowed metabolism, tear production. |
| **Happiness** | Increased dopamine and serotonin, relaxed muscles, improved digestion. |
| **Love & Affection** | Oxytocin release, reduced stress hormones, increased bonding behavior. |

◈ **Example:** When experiencing **anxiety**, the body releases **cortisol**, which increases alertness but, over time, can suppress the immune system if prolonged.

---

### 5. Emotional Memory and Conditioning

The **hippocampus and amygdala** store emotional memories, influencing how individuals respond to future situations.

- **Positive emotional memories** reinforce healthy responses (e.g., feeling joy when hearing a childhood song).

- **Negative emotional memories** can create trauma responses (e.g., anxiety triggered by past negative experiences).

◆ **Example:** A child bitten by a dog may develop **fear conditioning**, making them anxious around all dogs, even if they pose no threat.

---

### 6. Homoeopathic Perspective on Emotions

homoeopathy recognizes the deep connection between emotions and health. Certain remedies address emotional imbalances that manifest physically:

| Remedy | Indications |
|---|---|
| **Ignatia Amara** | For grief, suppressed emotions, mood swings. |
| **Natrum Muriaticum** | For long-standing sadness, bottled-up emotions, emotional withdrawal. |
| **Aurum Metallicum** | For deep depression, self-reproach, despair. |
| **Pulsatilla** | For emotional sensitivity, need for reassurance, weepiness. |
| **Staphysagria** | For suppressed anger, humiliation, emotional trauma. |

◆ **Example:** Someone dealing with unresolved grief may benefit from **Ignatia Amara**, which helps release emotional blockages.

---

### 7. Emotional Health and Disease Connection

Unresolved or extreme emotions contribute to the development of various diseases:

- **Chronic stress → High blood pressure, heart disease, digestive disorders.**
- **Unresolved grief → Depression, weakened immune function.**
- **Suppressed anger → Liver dysfunction, migraines, hypertension.**
- **Fear and anxiety → Adrenal exhaustion, hormonal imbalances.**

◈ **Example:** Studies have shown that prolonged emotional stress weakens the immune system, making individuals more susceptible to infections and chronic conditions.

---

### Conclusion

*Emotions are not just fleeting feelings but powerful forces that shape mental, physical, and even spiritual well-being. Understanding emotions from a neurological, physiological, and Homoeopathic perspective allows for* ***holistic emotional regulation****, leading to improved health and resilience.*

---

## Chapter 6: Evolution of Man and the History of Emotions

### Introduction

Emotions are not merely personal experiences but are deeply embedded in human evolution. They have played a crucial role in survival, social bonding, and adaptation throughout history. The evolution of emotions is intertwined with the biological and cultural evolution of humans, shaping how we perceive and respond to our environment.

This chapter explores how emotions evolved from primitive survival mechanisms to complex psychological experiences that influence modern human behaviour.

---

### 1. The Evolutionary Basis of Emotions

Emotions developed as adaptive responses to environmental challenges, helping early humans survive and thrive. The **basic emotions**—fear, anger, joy, sadness, and disgust—served specific survival purposes:

| Emotion | Evolutionary Purpose |
|---|---|
| **Fear** | Helped early humans escape predators and avoid danger. |
| **Anger** | Encouraged defence of territory, resources, and social status. |
| **Happiness** | Reinforced social bonding and cooperation. |
| **Sadness** | Encouraged reflection, support-seeking, and learning from losses. |
| **Disgust** | Prevented ingestion of harmful or spoiled food, aiding survival. |

◈ **Example:** Early humans who experienced fear in response to a predator were more likely to survive by fleeing or hiding, ensuring the continuation of their genetic line.

---

### 2. The Evolution of the Brain and Emotional Processing

The human brain has evolved in layers, each contributing to emotional processing:

**A. The Reptilian Brain (Primitive Emotions) – 500 Million Years Ago**

- The oldest part of the brain (brainstem and basal ganglia).
- Controls basic survival instincts such as fight-or-flight, hunger, and territoriality.
- Emotionally, it governs **fear, aggression, and dominance**.

**B. The Limbic System (Social and Emotional Evolution) – 200 Million Years Ago**

- The **amygdala, hippocampus, and hypothalamus** evolved to regulate emotions and memory.
- Helped early mammals develop social bonds and care for offspring.
- Allowed for **attachment, pleasure-seeking, and emotional memory**.

**C. The Neocortex (Complex Emotions and Rational Thought) – 2-3 Million Years Ago**

- The newest part of the brain, unique to primates and humans.
- Enabled **advanced problem-solving, empathy, and moral reasoning**.
- Allowed emotions to be regulated by logic, culture, and personal experiences.

◈ **Example:** Unlike reptiles, which act purely on instinct, humans can suppress aggression by reasoning through the consequences.

---

## 3. The History of Emotions in Human Societies

As human societies evolved, emotions became more complex and were shaped by cultural and social factors:

### A. Prehistoric Societies (Survival and Basic Social Bonds)

- Early humans relied on **fear and cooperation** to survive.
- **Emotional expressions** (e.g., facial expressions, body language) helped in communication before language developed.
- Joy was linked to successful hunting, mating, and survival of offspring.

### B. Ancient Civilizations (Religious and Moral Emotions)

- Emotions like **guilt, shame, pride, and love** became central to social structures.
- **Religious texts and moral codes** regulated emotions, encouraging self-control.
- **Philosophers like Aristotle and Confucius** explored emotions as part of human virtue and ethics.

◈ **Example:** Ancient Egyptian, Greek, and Hindu texts describe emotions as divine forces that influence human destiny.

### C. Medieval Period (Religious Control and Emotional Expression)

- Emotions were often linked to sin or virtue (e.g., **anger = wrath, love = divine**).
- The church and monarchy dictated emotional behavior through strict moral codes.

- Art and literature reflected deep emotional states, such as **romantic love, grief, and spiritual ecstasy**.

◈ **Example:** Courtly love in medieval Europe idealized **romantic emotions**, shaping modern concepts of love and relationships

**D. Renaissance and Enlightenment (Rationality vs. Emotion)**

- Philosophers like **Descartes and Locke** debated whether emotions should be controlled by reason.
- Science began exploring emotions biologically, linking them to the nervous system.
- Emotions were **expressed more openly in art, music, and literature**.

◈ **Example:** Shakespeare's plays deeply explored human emotions, from ambition (*Macbeth*) to jealousy (*Othello*).

**E. Industrial Revolution to Modern Era (Psychology and Emotional Intelligence)**

- The 19th century saw **psychological theories** on emotions (*Freud, Darwin, James-Lange theory*).
- The 20th century introduced **emotional intelligence (EQ)** as a key factor in personal success.
- In modern society, emotions are studied scientifically and managed through **therapy, mindfulness, and medication**.

◈ **Example:** Today, neuroscientists use **brain imaging** to study emotional responses and how they impact mental health.

---

#### 4. The Role of Emotions in Social Evolution

As humans evolved, emotions became essential for building **complex societies**:

- **Empathy** helped create cooperative groups, leading to civilization development.
- **Love and attachment** fostered long-term relationships and parental care.
- **Guilt and shame** ensured individuals adhered to social norms, promoting social harmony.
- **Anger and rebellion** played roles in societal change, revolutions, and justice movements.

◈ **Example:** The emotion of **patriotism** evolved to unify large groups, leading to the formation of nations.

---

#### 5. Homoeopathic Perspective on the Evolution of Emotions

homoeopathy recognizes the influence of **evolutionary emotional patterns** in disease manifestation. Some remedies that address deep-rooted emotional conditions include:

| Remedy | Indications Related to Evolutionary Emotional Patterns |
|---|---|
| **Aconitum Napellus** | Sudden fear, panic attacks (primitive fear response). |
| **Nux Vomica** | Irritability, competitive stress (modern societal pressures). |
| **Ignatia Amara** | Grief and heartbreak (emotional adaptation challenges). |
| **Lycopodium** | Fear of failure, lack of confidence (hierarchical |

| | |
|---|---|
| | social pressure). |
| **Staphysagria** | Suppressed anger, trauma from authority figures (societal conditioning). |

◈ **Example:** A person suffering from **panic attacks** may respond well to **Aconitum**, which aligns with the primitive survival fear response.

---

### Conclusion

*Emotions have evolved from simple survival instincts to deeply complex human experiences that shape culture, health, and society. Understanding this history helps in* ***managing emotions holistically****, incorporating modern science, psychology, and homoeopathy for emotional well-being.*

---

## Chapter 7: Social and Environmental Influences on Mind and Emotion

### Introduction

Human emotions and thought processes are not developed in isolation. They are shaped by the **social and environmental factors** we experience from birth to adulthood. Our interactions with family, peers, culture, society, economy, and even the physical environment influence our emotions, mental health, and behavioural patterns.

This chapter explores how different external factors contribute to emotional well-being or distress, shaping the psychological landscape of an individual.

---

### 1. The Role of Family in Emotional Development

Family plays a foundational role in shaping emotional responses and psychological resilience. From infancy, a child's first emotional experiences are based on interactions with parents and caregivers.

**A. Attachment Theory** (Bowlby & Ainsworth)

- Secure Attachment: Leads to emotional stability, confidence, and strong interpersonal relationships.
- Insecure Attachment: Can cause anxiety, difficulty trusting others, and emotional volatility.

◈ **Example:** A child raised in a loving, supportive home will likely develop a positive self-image and emotional security. In contrast, a neglected child may develop emotional insecurities or attachment issues.

**B. Parenting Styles and Their Impact on Emotions** (Baumrind's Model)

- **Authoritative Parenting:** Balanced discipline and warmth → leads to emotional intelligence and confidence.
- **Authoritarian Parenting:** Strict control, low warmth → can cause anxiety, rebellion, or low self-esteem.
- **Permissive Parenting:** High warmth, low discipline → may lead to impulsiveness and emotional instability.
- **Neglectful Parenting:** Lack of care → can result in depression, lack of emotional regulation.

◈ **Example:** A child whose emotions are acknowledged and validated learns to regulate feelings better than a child whose emotions are dismissed.

---

### 2. Peer Influence and Social Relationships

As individuals grow, friendships and social interactions become crucial in shaping emotions and personality.

#### A. Peer Pressure and Emotional Impact

- Positive Peer Influence: Encourages emotional growth, resilience, and self-esteem.
- Negative Peer Influence: Leads to stress, anxiety, and poor decision-making.

◈ **Example:** A teenager in a supportive friend circle may develop confidence, while one in a toxic group may experience self-doubt and depression.

#### B. Social Rejection and Emotional Pain

- The brain processes social rejection similarly to physical pain.
- Loneliness and isolation can lead to anxiety, depression, and emotional withdrawal.

◈ **Example:** Studies show that rejection activates the same neural pathways as physical injury, emphasizing its emotional impact.

---

### 3. Cultural Influences on Emotional Expression

Different cultures shape how people express and regulate emotions.

#### A. Individualistic vs. Collectivist Cultures

- **Individualistic Cultures** (e.g., USA, Western Europe):
    - Emphasize personal achievement, independence.

    - Encourage emotional expression and assertiveness.
- **Collectivist Cultures** (e.g., India, Japan, China):
    - Emphasize group harmony, interdependence.
    - Suppress emotions to maintain social balance.

◈ **Example:** In Japan, emotional restraint is valued, while in the US, open emotional expression is encouraged.

**B. Religious and Spiritual Influences**

- Religions often guide emotional responses through moral teachings.
- Practices like meditation, prayer, and rituals influence emotional well-being.

◈ **Example:** Mindfulness and meditation in Buddhism help manage emotions like anger and anxiety.

---

**4. The Impact of Society and Social Media on Emotions**

Modern society and digital platforms have reshaped emotional experiences.

**A. The Role of Social Norms and Expectations**

- Society dictates emotional standards (e.g., men should not cry, women should be nurturing).
- Breaking these norms can lead to emotional distress or liberation.

◈ **Example:** The stigma around male vulnerability can lead to emotional suppression and mental health issues.

### B. Social Media and Emotional Well-being

- **Positive Effects:** Connection, inspiration, emotional support.
- **Negative Effects:** Comparison, cyberbullying, unrealistic expectations.

◈ **Example:** Seeing curated "perfect" lives on social media can lead to anxiety and self-esteem issues.

---

## 5. Economic and Financial Influences on Emotions

Economic stability or instability directly impacts mental and emotional well-being.

### A. Financial Stress and Mental Health

- Unemployment, debt, or poverty can lead to anxiety, depression, and low self-worth.
- Economic uncertainty causes chronic stress, impacting relationships and cognitive function.

◈ **Example:** A person struggling with debt may experience constant worry, disturbed sleep, and irritability, affecting overall emotional health.

### B. Wealth and Emotional Stability

- While financial security provides comfort, excessive wealth can lead to emotional isolation or pressure to maintain status.
- Studies show happiness increases with income but plateaus after meeting basic needs.

◈ **Example:** A wealthy businessman may face emotional stress due to intense competition and expectations, while a middle-class worker with financial security may have better emotional balance.

**C. Economic Crises and Collective Psychological Impact**

- Recessions, inflation, or economic crashes increase stress at both individual and societal levels.
- Job loss and financial hardship create widespread emotional distress.

◈ **Example:** The COVID-19 pandemic led to mass unemployment, increasing depression and anxiety rates globally.

---

**6. Environmental Factors Affecting Emotions**

Physical surroundings also impact emotional health.

**A. Urban vs. Rural Living**

- **Urban Areas:** High stress, noise pollution, fast-paced life → leads to anxiety.
- **Rural Areas:** Closer to nature, slower lifestyle → promotes mental well-being.

◈ **Example:** Studies show people living near greenery experience lower stress levels.

**B. Climate and Seasonal Changes**

- Sunlight exposure boosts serotonin (happiness chemical).
- Seasonal Affective Disorder (SAD) occurs due to low sunlight in winter.

◈ **Example:** Higher depression rates in areas with long winters due to lack of sunlight.

### C. Childhood Environment and Trauma

- **Early exposure to abuse, neglect, or violence** can rewire the brain's emotional responses.
- Trauma often leads to chronic stress, PTSD, or emotional dysregulation.

◈ **Example:** A child witnessing domestic violence may develop anxiety and emotional instability later in life.

---

## 7. Homoeopathic Perspective on Social and Environmental Influences

Homoeopathy recognizes how social and environmental factors shape emotional health. Remedies can address emotions arising from external influences.

| Remedy | Indications |
|---|---|
| **Natrum Muriaticum** | Grief, suppressed emotions from social isolation or heartbreak. |
| **Ignatia Amara** | Emotional distress from rejection or loss. |
| **Lycopodium** | Low confidence due to strict societal expectations. |
| **Pulsatilla** | Emotional dependency influenced by environmental changes. |
| **Staphysagria** | Emotional suppression due to abuse or authority control. |

◈ **Example:** A person suffering from social anxiety due to past bullying may benefit from **Lycopodium** to restore confidence.

---

### Conclusion

*Social, environmental, and economic factors significantly impact emotional well-being. Understanding these influences allows us to manage emotions better and seek appropriate healing methods, whether through psychology, lifestyle changes, or Homoeopathic remedies.*

---

## Chapter 8:Interpersonal Relationships and Emotional Well-being

### Introduction

Human emotions are deeply influenced by interpersonal relationships. From birth to old age, our mental and emotional health is shaped by the relationships we form—with family, friends, romantic partners, colleagues, and society at large. Healthy relationships can provide emotional support, security, and happiness, whereas toxic or broken relationships can contribute to stress, anxiety, and emotional trauma.

In this chapter, we will explore the different aspects of interpersonal relationships, their impact on emotional well-being, and the role of homoeopathy in addressing emotional imbalances caused by relationship dynamics.

---

### 1. Types of Interpersonal Relationships

#### A. Familial Relationships

- **Parent-Child Relationships:** The first emotional bond formed, shaping an individual's attachment style and emotional regulation.

- **Sibling Bonds:** Can be sources of companionship, competition, or emotional conflict.
- **Extended Family:** Grandparents, aunts, uncles, and cousins contribute to social and emotional development.

◈ **Example:** A child raised in a nurturing family develops emotional security, while one in a neglectful family may struggle with self-worth.

**B. Friendships**

- Provide emotional support, companionship, and shared experiences.
- Healthy friendships boost self-esteem and emotional resilience.
- Toxic friendships can lead to stress, self-doubt, and emotional exhaustion.

◈ **Example:** A supportive friend helps navigate stress, while a toxic friend drains emotional energy.

**C. Romantic Relationships**

- Strong emotional connections that influence self-esteem, happiness, and personal growth.
- Healthy romantic relationships provide security and love.
- Unhealthy relationships can cause emotional distress and long-term psychological damage.

◈ **Example:** A secure partner fosters emotional stability, whereas an emotionally unavailable partner can lead to anxiety.

### D. Professional Relationships

- Impact self-esteem, motivation, and emotional well-being in the workplace.
- Healthy work relationships enhance job satisfaction and mental health.
- Workplace conflicts can lead to emotional distress and burnout.

◈ **Example:** A supportive manager encourages growth, while a toxic boss induces anxiety.

### E. Social and Community Relationships

- Interactions with Neighbors, acquaintances, and societal groups shape social identity.
- A strong community connection enhances emotional well-being.
- Social isolation can lead to loneliness and depression.

◈ **Example:** Being part of a supportive cultural or religious group provides a sense of belonging.

---

## 2. Emotional Communication in Relationships

Effective communication is essential for maintaining healthy relationships.

### A. Verbal Communication

- Honest and clear conversations build trust and reduce emotional stress.
- Miscommunication can lead to misunderstandings and conflicts.

◈ **Example:** Expressing concerns openly prevents resentment.

**B. Non-Verbal Communication**

- Body language, facial expressions, and tone of voice convey emotions.
- Misinterpreting non-verbal cues can lead to confusion.

◈ **Example:** A frown can indicate sadness or disapproval.

**C. Active Listening**

- Understanding and empathizing with others' emotions.
- Helps in resolving conflicts and strengthening emotional bonds.

◈ **Example:** A friend feeling heard and understood experiences emotional relief.

---

**3. Relationship Challenges and Emotional Impact**

**A. Conflict and Disagreements**

- Conflicts are natural but need to be resolved effectively.
- Poor conflict resolution leads to stress and emotional suppression.

◈ **Example:** A workplace disagreement handled through open communication fosters teamwork, while unresolved tension creates a toxic environment.

**B. Toxic Relationships**

- Emotional abuse, manipulation, or excessive control can cause psychological damage.
- Codependency can lead to emotional exhaustion.

◈ **Example:** A controlling partner may lead to low self-esteem and anxiety.

**C. Breakups, Divorce, and Loss**

- Endings of relationships cause emotional pain and distress.
- Healing requires emotional processing and self-care.

◈ **Example:** A person grieving a breakup may experience depression, which needs emotional support to recover.

**D. Social Rejection and Loneliness**

- The brain processes social rejection similarly to physical pain.
- Loneliness can contribute to anxiety and depression.

◈ **Example:** Repeated social rejection can lower self-esteem and increase emotional withdrawal.

---

**4. Psychological Theories of Interpersonal Relationships**

**A. Attachment Theory (Bowlby & Ainsworth)**

- **Secure Attachment:** Leads to emotional stability, confidence, and trust in relationships.
- **Insecure Attachment:** Causes anxiety, fear of abandonment, and difficulty forming healthy bonds.

**B. Love and Relationship Theories**

- **Sternberg's Triangular Theory of Love:** Consists of intimacy, passion, and commitment.

- **Five Love Languages (Gary Chapman):** Words of affirmation, quality time, physical touch, acts of service, and gifts.

### C. Social Exchange Theory

- Relationships are based on perceived benefits and costs.
- Healthy relationships maintain a balance between giving and receiving.

---

## 5. Homoeopathic Approach to Emotional Health in Relationships

Homoeopathy acknowledges the emotional distress caused by interpersonal relationship challenges. Remedies can help restore emotional balance.

| Remedy | Indications |
|---|---|
| **Natrum Muriaticum** | Grief, heartbreak, emotional suppression. |
| **Ignatia Amara** | Emotional distress from rejection or loss. |
| **Lycopodium** | Low confidence and social anxiety. |
| **Pulsatilla** | Emotional dependency and insecurity. |
| **Staphysagria** | Emotional suppression due to abuse or authority control. |

◈ **Example:** A person struggling with heartbreak may benefit from **Ignatia Amara** to ease emotional pain.

---

**6. Strategies for Building Healthy Relationships**

- **Develop Emotional Intelligence:** Recognize and regulate emotions.
- **Practice Empathy:** Understand others' feelings and perspectives.
- **Establish Boundaries:** Maintain healthy limits in relationships.
- **Foster Trust and Honesty:** Strengthen bonds through openness.
- **Seek Professional Help:** Therapy or counselling for relationship struggles.

◈ **Example:** Setting boundaries in friendships helps maintain emotional well-being.

---

### Conclusion

*Interpersonal relationships are essential to emotional well-being. Healthy relationships provide support and happiness, while toxic ones can lead to emotional distress. Understanding relationship dynamics, improving communication, and addressing emotional imbalances through homoeopathy can enhance overall mental and emotional health.*

---

## Chapter 9: Dreams and the Mind – The Subconscious Connection

### Introduction

Dreams serve as windows into the subconscious mind, revealing hidden emotions, unresolved conflicts, and deep-seated fears.

homoeopathy, with its holistic approach, considers dreams a vital part of case-taking, offering insights into a person's mental and emotional state. This chapter explores the psychological and Homoeopathic understanding of dreams and their connection to the mind.

---

**A. The Science of Dreams – Psychological Perspectives**

1. **Freud's Theory (Psychoanalytic Perspective)**
    - Dreams are the "royal road to the unconscious."
    - They reveal suppressed desires and unresolved conflicts.
    - Example: A person dreaming of falling may have anxiety about losing control in real life.
2. **Jung's Perspective (Archetypal and Collective Unconscious)**
    - Dreams contain symbols from the collective unconscious.
    - Archetypes like the "Shadow" or "Anima/Animus" manifest in dreams.
    - Example: Dreaming of a wise old man may symbolize inner wisdom or guidance.
3. **Modern Neuroscientific View**
    - Dreams are the brain's way of processing emotions and memories.
    - The limbic system (emotions) and prefrontal cortex (rationality) interact during dreaming.

- Example: Stress-related dreams often occur due to high cortisol levels.

---

**B. Types of Dreams and Their Psychological Impact**

1. **Recurring Dreams**
    - Indicate unresolved emotions or traumas.
    - Example: Repeatedly dreaming of being chased may signal deep-seated anxiety.
2. **Nightmares**
    - Reflect fears, stress, or past traumas.
    - Example: A person with PTSD may experience vivid, disturbing dreams.
3. **Lucid Dreams**
    - The dreamer is aware they are dreaming and may control the dream.
    - Often associated with heightened self-awareness and emotional regulation.
4. **Prophetic or Intuitive Dreams**
    - Dreams that seem to predict future events or reveal hidden truths.
    - Example: Some people report dreaming of an illness before diagnosis.

---

### C. Homoeopathic Understanding of Dreams

In homoeopathy, dreams are analyzed to determine a patient's **emotional state, subconscious fears, and personality traits**. Specific dream patterns often correlate with certain remedies.

#### 1. Dreams Indicating Grief and Loss

- Dreaming of deceased loved ones, funerals, or abandonment.
- Related remedies: **Ignatia Amara, Natrum Muriaticum**.
- Example: A person who suppresses grief yet dreams of crying may need Natrum Muriaticum.

#### 2. Dreams of Falling or Drowning

- Reflect insecurity, fear of failure, or lack of control.
- Related remedies: **Gelsemium, Argentum Nitricum**.
- Example: A student fearing an upcoming exam may dream of falling, indicating Gelsemium.

#### 3. Dreams of Snakes or Animals

- Snakes symbolize hidden fears, deception, or deep transformation.
- Related remedies: **Lachesis (jealousy, suppressed emotions), Naja (guilt, sorrow)**.
- Example: A person with repressed anger may frequently dream of attacking snakes, indicating Lachesis.

#### 4. Dreams of Flying or Elevation

- Indicate ambition, freedom, or spiritual growth.

- Related remedies: **Phosphorus (excitable, visionary), Cannabis Indica (euphoric, expanded awareness)**.

**5. Night Terrors and Fear-Based Dreams**

- Indicate deep anxieties, childhood traumas, or phobias.
- Related remedies: **Stramonium (dark fears, terror), Kali Bromatum (delusions, paranoia)**.
- Example: A child waking up screaming due to night terrors may benefit from Stramonium.

---

### D. The Role of Miasms in Dream Patterns

Each miasm has characteristic dream themes:

1. **Psoric Miasm** – Dreams of struggling, poverty, or endless effort (Sulphur, Arsenicum Album).
2. **Sycotic Miasm** – Dreams of hiding, guilt, or secretive activities (Thuja, Medorrhinum).
3. **Syphilitic Miasm** – Nightmares, destruction, or self-harm themes (Aurum Metallicum, Mercurius).
4. **Tubercular Miasm** – Dreams of travel, escape, or adventure (Tuberculinum, Phosphorus).

---

### E. Conclusion

*Dreams serve as a powerful diagnostic tool in homoeopathy, reflecting deep-seated emotions and subconscious conflicts. By analyzing dream patterns, homoeopaths can identify the underlying miasmatic tendencies and select the most appropriate remedy. Understanding dreams allows for a deeper approach to emotional healing, aligning the conscious and subconscious mind towards holistic well-being.*

---

# Chapter 10: The Mind and Sexuality

## Introduction

Sexuality is a fundamental aspect of human life, deeply connected to the mind. It is influenced by psychological, emotional, hormonal, and social factors, making it more than just a physical experience. This chapter explores the intricate relationship between the mind and sexuality, covering aspects such as psychological influences, emotional connections, hormonal regulation, and the role of the brain in sexual behaviour.

---

### 1. Psychological Aspects of Sexuality

Sexuality is not merely a biological function but an experience shaped by thoughts, emotions, and personal beliefs. The mind plays a critical role in defining one's sexual identity, preferences, and expressions.

- **Sexual Identity & Orientation:** One's sense of sexual identity and orientation is formed in the mind and influenced by personal experiences, cultural norms, and societal conditioning.
- **Body Image & Self-Esteem:** How one perceives their body significantly impacts sexual confidence and satisfaction.

- **Trauma & Sexuality:** Past experiences, including sexual trauma or abuse, can profoundly shape sexual behaviours, leading to fear, avoidance, or hypersexuality.
- **Fantasies & Desires:** The mind constructs sexual fantasies, which are shaped by personal experiences, exposure, and subconscious desires.

---

### 2. Emotional Influence on Sexuality

Emotions are deeply tied to sexual desire, performance, and fulfilment. Emotional well-being enhances sexual experiences, whereas emotional disturbances can lead to dysfunction.

- **Love & Attachment:** Emotional intimacy strengthens sexual connection and pleasure through deeper trust and vulnerability.
- **Stress & Anxiety:** High stress levels can suppress libido, cause erectile dysfunction, or lead to difficulty in arousal.
- **Guilt & Shame:** Cultural and religious beliefs may create feelings of guilt, leading to repression, avoidance, or anxiety around sex.
- **Depression & Sexual Health:** Depression can reduce libido and cause sexual dysfunction due to lower dopamine and serotonin levels.
- **Emotional Trauma:** Unresolved emotional wounds can create barriers to healthy sexual expression.

---

### 3. Hormonal Influence on Sexual Behaviour

The mind influences hormone production, which in turn affects sexual desire and function.

- **Testosterone & Libido:** Higher levels of testosterone (in both men and women) are linked to increased sexual desire and energy.
- **Oxytocin & Bonding:** Released during physical intimacy, oxytocin strengthens emotional bonds and enhances trust between partners.
- **Dopamine & Pleasure:** Dopamine plays a significant role in the reward system, making sexual activity pleasurable and reinforcing sexual behaviour.
- **Serotonin & Mood Regulation:** Higher serotonin levels can decrease sexual desire, while lower levels may increase impulsivity.
- **Cortisol & Stress:** Chronic stress increases cortisol levels, which can negatively impact sexual function and libido.

---

### 4. The Brain's Role in Sexual Arousal

The brain is the primary organ that processes sexual stimuli and generates responses. Different brain regions contribute to various aspects of sexual experience.

- **Limbic System:** Comprising the amygdala, hypothalamus, and hippocampus, this system plays a key role in sexual desire and response.
- **Prefrontal Cortex:** This area regulates impulse control, decision-making, and emotional responses, influencing sexual behaviour.

- **Mirror Neurons & Desire:** Observing sexual stimuli or engaging in intimate touch activates mirror neurons, enhancing arousal.
- **Hypothalamus & Hormonal Regulation:** The hypothalamus regulates hormone release, which directly impacts libido and sexual function.

---

### 5. Subconscious Influences on Sexuality

Sexual desires and behaviours are often influenced by subconscious thoughts and past experiences.

- **Repressed Desires:** Social conditioning may suppress certain sexual desires, leading to internal conflicts.
- **Dreams & Sexuality:** Erotic dreams reflect subconscious sexual desires and unresolved emotional conflicts.
- **Freudian Perspective:** Sigmund Freud emphasized the role of unconscious desires in shaping sexual behaviours.
- **Cultural and Familial Influence:** Early childhood experiences and cultural conditioning shape attitudes toward sexuality.

---

### 6. Sexual Disorders and Psychological Causes

Many sexual disorders have psychological origins, highlighting the strong mind-body connection.

- **Erectile Dysfunction (ED):** Often linked to performance anxiety, depression, or past trauma.

- **Hypoactive Sexual Desire Disorder (HSDD):** Characterized by low sexual desire due to stress, hormonal imbalances, or emotional repression.
- **Premature Ejaculation:** Can be caused by anxiety, past experiences, or conditioned responses.
- **Sexual Aversion Disorder:** Develops due to trauma, negative experiences, or deep-seated fears about sexuality.

---

### 7. Healing the Mind-Sex Connection

Addressing mental and emotional blocks can significantly improve sexual well-being.

- **Therapeutic Approaches:** Cognitive-behavioural therapy (CBT), psychoanalysis, and sex therapy help in resolving sexual concerns.
- **Mindfulness & Meditation:** These practices enhance body awareness and improve sexual responsiveness.
- **Communication & Emotional Intimacy:** Open communication between partners fosters trust and enhances sexual satisfaction.
- **Homoeopathic Approach:** Remedies such as Lycopodium, Natrum Mur, and Staphysagria are used for treating psychological and emotional blocks affecting sexuality.

---

### Conclusion

*The link between the mind and sexuality is undeniable, shaping every aspect of sexual function and experience. Understanding this connection allows for a more holistic approach to sexual well-being, integrating psychological, emotional, and physiological aspects. By addressing mental barriers and enhancing emotional health, one can cultivate a fulfilling and balanced sexual life.*

---

# Chapter 11-: The Mind-Body Connection – A Physiological Perspective

## Introduction

The intricate link between the mind and body has been a subject of study in philosophy, psychology, and medicine for centuries. Modern neuroscience and physiology confirm that emotions, thoughts, and mental states directly influence physiological processes, shaping overall health and well-being. The mind is not separate from the body; rather, it communicates through complex networks of neurotransmitters, hormones, and neural circuits.

This chapter explores the physiological mechanisms by which the mind and emotions affect the body, emphasizing their role in maintaining homeostasis, influencing organ functions, and shaping human behaviour.

---

### 1. The Brain as the Central Processing Unit

The brain serves as the command center, processing emotions, thoughts, and sensory information while regulating bodily functions through the nervous and endocrine systems.

### A. Key Brain Structures Involved in Mind-Body Interaction

1. **Cerebral Cortex** – Responsible for higher cognitive functions, reasoning, and decision-making.

2. **Limbic System** – The emotional hub of the brain, including:
    - **Amygdala** – Processes emotions such as fear and pleasure.
    - **Hippocampus** – Involved in memory formation and emotional regulation.
    - **Hypothalamus** – Links the nervous system to the endocrine system, controlling bodily functions like temperature, hunger, and stress responses.
3. **Brainstem** – Regulates automatic functions such as heart rate and respiration.
4. **Prefrontal Cortex** – Involved in emotional control, impulse regulation, and rational thinking.

---

### 2. The Nervous System: The Highway Between Mind and Body

The nervous system is the primary communication channel linking the mind and body, comprising two main divisions:

**A. Central Nervous System (CNS)**

- Composed of the brain and spinal cord.
- Processes emotions and thoughts, triggering physiological responses.

**B. Peripheral Nervous System (PNS)**

- Connects the CNS to organs and muscles.
- Divided into:

1. **Somatic Nervous System** – Controls voluntary movements.
2. **Autonomic Nervous System (ANS)** – Regulates involuntary functions.
    - **Sympathetic Nervous System (SNS):** Activates fight-or-flight response.
    - **Parasympathetic Nervous System (PNS):** Promotes relaxation and recovery.

◈ **Example:** When facing danger, the **SNS** increases heart rate and dilates pupils, while the **PNS** helps the body relax after the threat is gone.

---

### 3. The Endocrine System: The Chemical Messenger

Emotions influence the endocrine system, which regulates hormones that affect various physiological functions.

#### A. Major Hormones Influencing Mind-Body Interaction

| Hormone | Function | Effect of Emotional States |
| --- | --- | --- |
| **Cortisol** | Stress response, metabolism | Chronic stress increases cortisol, leading to health issues. |
| **Adrenaline (Epinephrine)** | Fight-or-flight activation | Enhances alertness but prolonged secretion causes anxiety. |
| **Dopamine** | Pleasure, motivation | Low levels lead to depression; high levels contribute to addiction. |

| | | |
|---|---|---|
| **Serotonin** | Mood regulation | Deficiency linked to depression and anxiety. |
| **Oxytocin** | Bonding, trust | Promotes social bonding and emotional security. |
| **Endorphins** | Natural painkillers | Released during exercise, reducing stress and enhancing mood. |

◈ **Example:** A person experiencing long-term stress has elevated **cortisol**, which can weaken the immune system and cause fatigue.

---

### 4. Physiological Effects of Emotional States

Emotions directly impact bodily functions, influencing health and behaviour.

#### A. Stress and Its Impact

- Activates the **hypothalamic-pituitary-adrenal (HPA) axis**.
- Increases heart rate, blood pressure, and muscle tension.
- Chronic stress leads to **weakened immunity**, digestive issues, and cardiovascular problems.

◈ **Example:** Exam anxiety can cause digestive issues like nausea or diarrhea due to stress-induced activation of the gut-brain axis.

#### B. Fear and Anxiety Response

- Triggers **amygdala** and **sympathetic nervous system**.
- Increases **adrenaline** and **cortisol** levels.
- Symptoms include rapid heartbeat, sweating, and shallow breathing.

◈ **Example:** A person encountering a snake experiences rapid breathing and increased alertness due to an adrenaline surge.

### C. Happiness and Relaxation Effects

- Activates the **parasympathetic nervous system**.
- Increases **dopamine, serotonin, and oxytocin**.
- Promotes muscle relaxation, stable heart rate, and better digestion.

◈ **Example:** Laughing with friends releases endorphins, reducing stress and boosting immunity.

### D. Sadness and Depression

- Reduces **dopamine and serotonin levels**.
- Lowers energy levels and weakens immune response.
- Disrupts sleep patterns and appetite regulation.

◈ **Example:** A person grieving may experience fatigue, loss of appetite, and sleep disturbances.

---

## 5. The Gut-Brain Connection

The digestive system and brain communicate via the **vagus nerve** and the **gut microbiome**, influencing emotional health.

### A. Role of the Gut Microbiome

- Produces neurotransmitters like **serotonin** (90% of which is found in the gut).
- Imbalances in gut bacteria contribute to mood disorders.

◈ **Example:** An unhealthy diet leading to gut dysbiosis can result in anxiety and depression.

**B. Stress and Digestive Function**

- Acute stress slows digestion; chronic stress leads to disorders like IBS (Irritable Bowel Syndrome).

◈ **Example:** A person with work-related stress may experience frequent indigestion or stomach ulcers.

---

### 6. Sleep and Its Role in Mind-Body Balance

Sleep is essential for cognitive function, emotional regulation, and physical health.

**A. Sleep Cycle and Brain Function**

- **Non-REM Sleep:** Body repair and immune strengthening.
- **REM Sleep:** Emotional processing and memory consolidation.

**B. Effects of Sleep Deprivation**

- Increases **cortisol**, leading to stress and anxiety.
- Reduces **dopamine and serotonin**, contributing to mood disorders.

◈ **Example:** Chronic sleep deprivation can impair decision-making and increase emotional instability.

---

### 7. The Role of Exercise in Mind-Body Integration

Physical activity influences mental health by:

- Increasing **endorphins and dopamine**, enhancing mood.
- Reducing stress hormones like **cortisol**.

- Improving cognitive function and memory.

◈ **Example:** Regular exercise reduces anxiety and boosts self-esteem through neurochemical balance.

---

### Conclusion

*The mind and body are deeply interconnected, communicating through the nervous, endocrine, and immune systems. Emotions and thoughts influence physical health, and physiological states impact mental well-being. Understanding these mechanisms is crucial for maintaining a balanced and healthy life.*

---

## Chapter 12: Mind and Organ-Wise Connection

### Introduction

Different emotions and mental states influence specific organs and their physiological responses. Understanding these connections helps us recognize how emotional well-being impacts physical health and vice versa.

---

### A. Brain and Heart Connection

- Stress and anxiety increase heart rate and blood pressure via the **sympathetic nervous system**.
- Chronic emotional distress may contribute to heart disease and hypertension.
- Positive emotions stimulate **parasympathetic activity**, lowering heart rate and promoting cardiovascular health.

◈ **Example:** Chronic worry can lead to hypertension, whereas deep breathing and meditation can reduce heart rate and improve heart function.

---

**B. Mind and Digestive System**

- The **gut-brain axis** links emotions with digestion through neural and biochemical pathways.
- Stress affects gut motility, causing issues like **acid reflux, bloating, or irritable bowel syndrome (IBS)**.
- Gut microbiota influences mood by producing neurotransmitters like **serotonin**.

◈ **Example:** A person experiencing stage fright may have sudden diarrhoea due to stress-induced activation of the gut.

---

**C. Mind and Respiratory System**

- Anxiety can lead to **shallow breathing or hyperventilation**.
- Stress-related respiratory changes affect **oxygen levels and lung function**.
- Mindful breathing techniques can regulate the respiratory rate and improve oxygenation.

◈ **Example:** A person experiencing a panic attack may hyperventilate, causing dizziness and chest tightness.

---

**D. Mind and Muscular System**

- Emotional tension causes **muscle stiffness and pain**, especially in the neck, shoulders, and lower back.
- Chronic stress can lead to conditions like **fibromyalgia**.
- Relaxation techniques help reduce **muscle tension and improve flexibility**.

◈ **Example:** A person under prolonged stress may develop **tension headaches** due to tight neck muscles.

---

**E. Mind and Skin**

- Emotional states influence skin health through **stress hormones**.
- Anxiety and stress can trigger **acne, psoriasis, or eczema**.
- Positive emotions promote **better circulation and a healthy glow**.

◈ **Example:** A student experiencing exam stress may develop **acne breakouts** due to increased cortisol levels.

---

**F. Mind and Immune System**

- Chronic stress weakens the **immune system**, increasing susceptibility to infections.
- Positive emotions enhance **immune responses**, promoting better health.

◈ **Example:** Long-term grief can reduce immunity, making a person prone to **colds and flu**.

### G. Mind and Kidney Function

- The kidneys are affected by **chronic stress, anxiety, and fear**, which can alter fluid balance and blood pressure.
- Prolonged emotional distress can increase **cortisol and adrenaline**, leading to increased strain on the kidneys.
- Fear and anxiety are traditionally linked to kidney function in holistic medicine, suggesting a deep psychosomatic connection.
- Chronic stress may contribute to kidney disease by causing **high blood pressure and metabolic imbalances**.

◈ **Example:** A person dealing with chronic fear or anxiety may develop **frequent urination or kidney-related disorders** due to prolonged activation of the stress response.

---

### Conclusion

*The intricate relationship between the mind and various organs demonstrates how emotions and mental states influence overall health. Recognizing these connections can help in managing stress, improving well-being, and preventing chronic health conditions.*

---

## Chapter 13: Emotional Patterns and Chronic Diseases

### Introduction

Emotions play a fundamental role in shaping human health. When negative emotional patterns persist over time, they create physiological imbalances, leading to chronic diseases. Understanding how specific emotional states contribute to different illnesses helps in both prevention and holistic healing.

---

### A. Stress and Its Role in Chronic Diseases

- Chronic stress disrupts the balance of the autonomic nervous system and the endocrine system.
- Leads to elevated cortisol levels, increasing inflammation and reducing immune function.
- Associated with hypertension, diabetes, heart disease, and autoimmune disorders.

◈ **Example:** A person experiencing prolonged work-related stress may develop high blood pressure, eventually leading to cardiovascular issues.

---

### B. Anxiety and Cardiovascular Disorders

- Persistent anxiety triggers excessive sympathetic nervous system activation.
- Increases heart rate, blood pressure, and risk of arrhythmias.
- Long-term anxiety is linked to heart disease, stroke, and chronic fatigue.

◈ **Example:** A person suffering from generalized anxiety disorder may have frequent palpitations and an increased risk of developing hypertension.

---

### C. Depression and Metabolic Disorders

- Depression alters neurotransmitter levels, affecting metabolism and digestion.
- Can lead to weight gain, insulin resistance, and Type 2 diabetes.
- Depressed individuals often adopt unhealthy lifestyles, worsening their condition.

◈ **Example:** A person struggling with chronic sadness may develop emotional eating habits, leading to obesity and diabetes.

---

### D. Suppressed Emotions and Autoimmune Diseases

- Repressed emotions create internal stress, weakening immune function.
- Emotional suppression is linked to rheumatoid arthritis, lupus, and multiple sclerosis.
- Chronic unresolved grief or anger can trigger inflammatory responses in the body.

◈ **Example:** A person suppressing anger for years may develop rheumatoid arthritis due to persistent inflammation.

---

### E. Fear and Kidney Disorders

- Fear stimulates adrenaline and cortisol release, impacting kidney function.
- Chronic fear can lead to high blood pressure, fluid imbalances, and kidney disease.

- Traditional medicine associates fear with kidney weakness, emphasizing emotional health.

◈ **Example:** A person constantly living in fear due to financial insecurity may develop chronic kidney issues.

---

**F. Guilt and Digestive Disorders**

- Guilt affects digestion by altering gut motility and enzyme secretion.
- Linked to irritable bowel syndrome (IBS), gastritis, and acid reflux.
- The gut-brain axis plays a key role in processing emotions.

◈ **Example:** Someone carrying long-term guilt may experience frequent stomach ulcers due to excess acid production.

---

**G. Loneliness and Neurodegenerative Diseases**

- Social isolation contributes to cognitive decline and dementia.
- Chronic loneliness increases stress hormones, leading to brain inflammation.
- Meaningful social connections help maintain cognitive function.

◈ **Example:** Elderly individuals with limited social interaction have a higher risk of developing Alzheimer's disease.

---

### Conclusion

*Chronic emotional patterns shape disease development over time. Identifying and addressing negative emotions is crucial for preventing and managing chronic illnesses. Holistic approaches, including lifestyle changes, therapy, and homoeopathy, can help restore emotional and physical health.*

---

## Chapter 14: Subconscious Emotions and Their Manifestation in Physical Health and Disease Patterns

### Introduction

### A. Understanding the Subconscious Mind

The subconscious mind operates beneath conscious awareness, storing emotions, memories, and unresolved conflicts. It plays a vital role in shaping our physical health, as emotional imprints from past experiences influence bodily functions. Unresolved subconscious emotions can manifest as chronic illnesses, autoimmune disorders, and even structural abnormalities in the body.

### B. The Mind-Body Connection: Pathways of Influence

The link between subconscious emotions and physical health is mediated through various physiological systems:

1. **The Autonomic Nervous System (ANS)** – Regulates involuntary functions such as heart rate, digestion, and immune response. Stressful subconscious emotions activate the sympathetic nervous system, leading to chronic inflammation and disease.

2. **The Endocrine System** – Emotional suppression affects hormonal balance, leading to conditions such as thyroid disorders, adrenal fatigue, and metabolic syndromes.
3. **The Immune System** – Emotional distress weakens immunity, making the body susceptible to infections, autoimmune diseases, and cancer.

---

### C. How Subconscious Emotions Influence Specific Diseases

#### 1. Cardiovascular Diseases (Heart and Circulatory System)

- Suppressed grief and emotional repression contribute to hypertension and heart disease.
- Chronic stress leads to increased cortisol levels, damaging arteries.
- **Example:** Individuals with unresolved emotional trauma often experience recurrent palpitations, high blood pressure, or angina.

#### 2. Gastrointestinal Disorders (Digestive System)

- Anxiety and suppressed fear disrupt gut motility, causing irritable bowel syndrome (IBS), acid reflux, and ulcers.
- The gut-brain axis shows that subconscious stress alters gut microbiota.
- **Example:** A person holding onto childhood fear may develop chronic gastritis or ulcerative colitis.

#### 3. Respiratory Diseases (Lungs and Breathing Patterns)

- Unexpressed grief and emotional suffocation manifest as asthma, bronchitis, or chronic respiratory conditions.

- **Example:** Asthmatic patients often have a history of emotional suppression, especially related to loss or abandonment.

**4. Autoimmune Disorders**

- Chronic emotional self-attack (guilt, self-rejection) can lead to conditions like lupus, rheumatoid arthritis, and multiple sclerosis.
- **Example:** A person who internalizes guilt and self-blame may develop Hashimoto's thyroiditis or fibromyalgia.

**5. Skin Disorders (Psoriasis, Eczema, and Acne)**

- Emotional distress leads to inflammatory skin conditions due to excessive cortisol production.
- **Example:** Individuals who suppress anger often experience recurrent acne breakouts or eczema flare-ups.

**6. Chronic Pain and Musculoskeletal Disorders**

- Emotional repression results in chronic tension, leading to migraines, back pain, and fibromyalgia.
- **Example:** A person carrying emotional burdens from childhood may develop persistent lower back pain.

---

### D. The Role of Miasms in Disease Formation

Miasmatic tendencies further explain how subconscious emotions contribute to disease patterns:

1. **Psoric Miasm** – Anxiety, insecurity, and self-doubt leading to skin diseases, allergies, and digestive issues.

2. **Sycotic Miasm** – Suppressed guilt and emotional hiding manifesting as growths, tumours, and metabolic disorders.
3. **Syphilitic Miasm** – Deep-seated trauma and destructive emotions contributing to autoimmune diseases and neurological disorders.
4. **Tubercular Miasm** – Restlessness and emotional dissatisfaction leading to respiratory and bone diseases.

---

### E. Healing Subconscious Emotional Patterns

Healing requires awareness and conscious effort to release emotional blockages:

1. **Homoeopathic Remedies** – Individualized remedies like Ignatia, Natrum Muriaticum, and Staphysagria help process and release emotional imprints.
2. **Meditation and Mindfulness** – Aids in recognizing and transforming subconscious emotional patterns.
3. **Psychotherapy and Emotional Release Techniques** – Techniques like hypnotherapy, EFT (Emotional Freedom Technique), and journaling help resolve suppressed emotions.

---

### F. Conclusion

*Subconscious emotions play a profound role in shaping physical health and disease patterns. By addressing emotional imprints and applying holistic healing approaches, it is possible to prevent and even reverse many chronic conditions.*

---

## Chapter 15: homoeopathy and the Mind – Insights from Hahnemann, Kent, and Other Masters

### Introduction

Homoeopathy, as a holistic system of medicine, recognizes the intricate connection between the mind and body. The emotional and mental state of a person plays a pivotal role in disease development and healing. This chapter explores the Homoeopathic understanding of the mind as conceptualized by Samuel Hahnemann, James Tyler Kent, and other prominent homoeopaths, with a focus on miasmatic influences on the mind.

---

### A. Hahnemann's View on Mind and Disease

- Samuel Hahnemann, the founder of homoeopathy, emphasized the role of the **vital force** in maintaining health.
- He recognized that mental and emotional states are central to disease progression and healing.
- He observed that some diseases begin with mental disturbances before leading to physical symptoms, reinforcing the modern psychosomatic concept.
- In the "Organon of Medicine," particularly in **Aphorism 9**, he stated that the "spirit-like vital force" governs life and is responsible for health or disease.
- Hahnemann proposed that diseases arise due to disturbances in the *vital force* (Lebenskraft), which is an immaterial energy governing the body.
- Mental and emotional states strongly influence this vital force, leading to either health or illness.

- In *Organon of Medicine*, aphorism §210-230, he highlights that mental and emotional factors play a primary role in disease manifestation.
- **Mental symptoms** are considered the most crucial indicators for remedy selection.

◈ **Example:** In cases of chronic disease, a homoeopath prioritizes mental and emotional symptoms over physical ones when choosing a remedy.

---

**B. Kent's Contribution – The Mind as the Center of Disease**

- James Tyler Kent, a major contributor to Homoeopathic philosophy, expanded on Hahnemann's ideas by asserting that disease primarily originates in the **mind and emotions**.
- He categorized remedies based on **constitutional types**, emphasizing the importance of mental and emotional characteristics.
- Kent believed that if mental symptoms were not addressed, physical symptoms would persist or return.
- He introduced the **hierarchy of symptoms**, where mental symptoms hold the highest rank.

◈ **Example:** A patient with deep-seated grief may need **Natrum Muriaticum**, even if their physical complaints seem unrelated.

---

### C. Contributions of Other Homoeopathic Masters

#### 1. Dr. Constantine Hering – The Father of American homoeopathy

- Hering developed **Hering's Law of Cure**, which states that healing progresses from **inside out, from more vital organs to less vital ones, and in reverse order of symptom appearance**.
- He emphasized that **emotional and mental healing precedes physical healing**.
- He also stressed the importance of studying dreams, fears, and subconscious patterns in remedy selection.

◈ **Example:** A person undergoing Homoeopathic treatment may first experience an emotional release before physical symptoms improve.

#### 2. Dr. John Henry Clarke – Deep Miasmatic Understanding

- Clarke expanded on **miasmatic theory**, emphasizing how inherited miasms influence mental states.
- He classified constitutional types based on **mental, emotional, and hereditary tendencies**.
- His materia medica provides detailed psychological profiles of Homoeopathic remedies.

◈ **Example:** A child with an inherited **sycotic miasm** may exhibit **deep-seated fears, secretiveness, and compulsive behavior**, requiring a remedy like **Medorrhinum**.

---

**D. Miasms and Their Influence on the Mind**

Hahnemann introduced the concept of **miasms**, which are inherited or acquired tendencies toward chronic diseases. Each miasm manifests with specific mental and emotional traits.

**1. Psora – The Miasm of Anxiety and Deficiency**

- Characterized by **worry, insecurity, and hypersensitivity**.
- Patients often suffer from **anxiety, fear of poverty, and anticipatory nervousness**.
- Mental restlessness and overthinking are common.
- Remedies: **Arsenicum Album, Sulphur, Calcarea Carbonica**.

◈ **Example:** A person constantly worrying about the future and financial stability may need **Arsenicum Album**.

**2. Sycosis – The Miasm of Excess and Suppression**

- Associated with **pride, jealousy, and obsessive tendencies**.
- Patients may have **fears of humiliation, compulsive behaviors, and secretiveness**.
- Suppressed emotions often lead to physical ailments like tumors or warts.
- Remedies: **Thuja, Medorrhinum, Natrum Sulphuricum**.

◈ **Example:** A person with an obsessive fear of being judged, leading to social withdrawal, may require **Thuja**.

**3. Syphilis – The Miasm of Destruction and Despair**

- Linked with **deep depression, suicidal tendencies, and destructive behaviors**.

- Patients may experience **paranoia, guilt, and severe mental agony**.
- It is associated with self-destructive habits and severe mental distress.
- Remedies: **Aurum Metallicum, Mercurius, Lachesis**.

◈ **Example:** A person suffering from **intense guilt and suicidal thoughts** may benefit from **Aurum Metallicum**.

**4. Tubercular Miasm – The Miasm of Restlessness and Dissatisfaction**

- Marked by **impulsiveness, desire for change, and frustration**.
- Patients may be **idealistic yet restless, frequently shifting goals**.
- Can lead to nervous exhaustion and a sense of constant dissatisfaction.
- Remedies: **Tuberculinum, Phosphorus, Calcarea Phosphorica**.

◈ **Example:** A highly ambitious but easily frustrated individual may need **Tuberculinum**.

---

### E. Homoeopathic Approach to Mental and Emotional Healing

- homoeopathy treats the **individual as a whole**, considering emotional, mental, and physical aspects.
- **Remedies are selected based on constitutional type and mental state** rather than just physical symptoms.

- **Dreams, fears, anxieties, and emotional patterns** are all analyzed during remedy selection.

◆ **Example:** A patient with a history of deep-seated grief who prefers solitude and is emotionally closed off might need **Ignatia Amara**.

---

### F. Conclusion

*Homoeopathy offers a unique and profound understanding of the mind and its connection to health. Hahnemann laid the foundation for mind-body healing, while Kent, Hering, and Clarke expanded on it, emphasizing the central role of emotions and miasms in chronic diseases. By treating mental and emotional symptoms, homoeopathy aims to bring deep and lasting healing.*

---

## Chapter 16: Case Taking According to Psychodynamic Evaluations

### Introduction

### A. Psychodynamic Case Taking in homoeopathy

Psychodynamic case taking integrates deep psychological understanding with classical Homoeopathic principles. It focuses on uncovering subconscious emotions, defence mechanisms, and early life experiences that shape the individual's current health state. This approach helps in selecting the most accurate remedy by identifying the root causes of physical and mental ailments.

---

### B. Key Components of Psychodynamic Case Taking

#### 1. Early Life Experiences and Emotional Imprints

- Understanding childhood traumas, parental influences, and significant emotional events.
- Exploring how these experiences contribute to personality development and disease patterns.
- **Example:** A person with a history of emotional neglect may develop deep insecurity and chronic anxiety-related disorders.

#### 2. Defence Mechanisms and Coping Strategies

- Identifying psychological defence mechanisms like repression, denial, projection, or displacement.
- Understanding how these mechanisms influence disease progression.
- **Example:** A patient with chronic headaches may suppress anger and express it through somatic symptoms.

#### 3. The Unconscious Mind and Symbolism

- Dreams, fears, and symbolic expressions provide insight into subconscious conflicts.
- Recurring thoughts, nightmares, and obsessive behaviours often reveal unresolved emotional wounds.
- **Example:** A patient with nightmares of drowning may have unresolved trauma linked to emotional suffocation in childhood.

#### 4. Emotional and Behavioural Patterns

- Analyzing the patient's predominant emotional reactions (e.g., fear, guilt, grief, anger, sadness).
- Observing repeated behavioural cycles in relationships and social interactions.
- **Example:** A patient with recurrent depression may have a pattern of self-sabotage stemming from deep-seated guilt.

#### 5. Miasmatic Influence in Psychodynamic Case Taking

- **Psoric Miasm:** Anxiety, insecurity, fear of failure.
- **Sycotic Miasm:** Suppressed emotions, secrecy, hidden fears.
- **Syphilitic Miasm:** Destructive tendencies, deep despair, suicidal thoughts.
- **Tubercular Miasm:** Restlessness, dissatisfaction, need for escape.

---

### C. Step-by-Step Approach to Psychodynamic Case Taking

#### Step 1: Establishing Rapport and Trust

- Creating a safe space for the patient to express emotions without fear of judgment.
- Using open-ended questions to encourage free expression.

#### Step 2: Exploring Presenting Complaints in Depth

- Understanding the emotional context of symptoms.
- Identifying any patterns between symptoms and emotional states.

**Step 3: Delving into Past Emotional Traumas**

- Investigating past losses, childhood fears, and significant emotional events.
- Recognizing unresolved grief or suppressed emotions.

**Step 4: Analyzing Relationship Dynamics**

- Assessing interactions with family, partners, friends, and colleagues.
- Identifying patterns of dependency, control, or emotional isolation.

**Step 5: Identifying Core Mental and Emotional Rubrics**

- Matching psychological traits with Homoeopathic remedies.
- Example: **Natrum Muriaticum** (grief, suppressed emotions), **Lachesis** (jealousy, loquacity), **Stramonium** (fear of darkness, night terrors).

---

**D. Practical Example of Psychodynamic Case Taking**

**Case Example:** A 35-year-old woman presents with chronic migraines and anxiety.

- **Early Life:** Grew up in a strict household, emotionally suppressed.
- **Defense Mechanism:** Represses anger, avoids confrontation.
- **Dreams:** Often dreams of being trapped, unable to escape.
- **Behavioral Patterns:** Overworks herself, struggles with self-worth.

- **Miasmatic Influence:** Sycotic (hidden emotions, fear of exposure).
- **Possible Remedy: Staphysagria** (suppressed anger, perfectionism, resentment).

---

### E. Conclusion

*Psychodynamic case taking in homoeopathy provides a deeper understanding of the patient's subconscious mind, emotional imprints, and behavioural patterns. By integrating this approach, homoeopaths can prescribe remedies that address the true root of the disease, leading to profound and lasting healing.*

---

## Chapter 17: Homoeopathic Case Taking Questionnaire – A Detailed Approach

### Introduction

### A. Homoeopathic Case Taking

Homoeopathic case taking is a deep and holistic process that helps identify the root cause of disease by understanding the patient's physical, emotional, and mental state. A well-structured questionnaire aids in gathering comprehensive information essential for prescribing the most suitable remedy.

---

### B. General Patient Information

1. **Name:**
2. **Age & Date of Birth:**
3. **Gender:**

4. **Occupation:**
5. **Marital Status & Relationship Details:**
6. **Chief Complaints (in order of priority):**
7. **Duration of Complaints:**
8. **Past Medical History:**
9. **Family Medical History (hereditary tendencies):**
10. **Any Major Surgery or Hospitalization:**

---

## C. Psychodynamic Analysis & Mind-Emotion Relationship

### 1. Mind & Personality

- How do you describe your personality (introvert, extrovert, sensitive, aggressive, etc.)?
- How do you handle stress and pressure?
- Any persistent fears or phobias (darkness, heights, loneliness, etc.)?
- Do you have repetitive thoughts or compulsions?
- Do you experience mood swings? If yes, what triggers them?
- Any history of past trauma or emotional distress?
- How do you react to criticism or rejection?

### 2. Emotional Responses

- How do you express anger? (Suppressed, aggressive, passive-aggressive, etc.)

- Do you cry easily? If so, what triggers it?
- Do you experience jealousy, possessiveness, or excessive attachment?
- How do you deal with grief and loss?
- Any recurring dreams or nightmares?
- What emotions do you suppress the most and why?
- How do you handle disappointment and failure?

**3. Relationship Dynamics & Social Behaviour**

- How is your relationship with family, friends, and colleagues?
- Do you feel dependent on others emotionally, or do you prefer isolation?
- How do you handle conflicts and disagreements?
- Any unresolved past relationship trauma?
- How do you express love and affection?
- Do you struggle with trust issues in relationships?

**4. Subconscious Influences & Symbolism**

- Any significant dreams that repeat frequently? What emotions do they evoke?
- Are there any specific childhood fears that still affect you?
- Do you have unexplained physical symptoms with no medical cause?
- Have you ever noticed physical ailments triggered by specific emotional experiences?

- How does your body react to strong emotions (e.g., stomach ache, headaches, palpitations)?

**5. Emotional Impact on Physical Health**

- Do you experience anxiety-related symptoms (shortness of breath, palpitations, sweating)?
- Have you noticed any correlation between emotions and digestive issues?
- Do stressful situations trigger headaches or muscle pain?
- How do emotional states affect your energy levels (fatigue, hyperactivity, sluggishness)?
- Have you experienced skin conditions worsening during stress or emotional upheaval?

**6. Miasmatic Influence in Emotional Health**

- **Psoric Miasm:** Anxiety, insecurity, fear of failure.
- **Sycotic Miasm:** Suppressed emotions, secrecy, hidden fears.
- **Syphilitic Miasm:** Destructive tendencies, deep despair, suicidal thoughts.
- **Tubercular Miasm:** Restlessness, dissatisfaction, need for escape.

---

**D. Physical General Symptoms**

**1. Sleep Patterns**

- How many hours do you sleep on average?

- Do you suffer from insomnia, disturbed sleep, or vivid dreams?
- Any particular sleeping position preference?

**2. Appetite & Cravings**

- How is your appetite – normal, increased, decreased?
- Do you have specific food cravings (sweet, salty, spicy, sour)?
- Any food aversions?
- Do you have food allergies?
- Do you experience indigestion, bloating, or acidity?

**3. Thirst & Water Intake**

- How much water do you drink daily?
- Do you prefer cold or warm drinks?

**4. Temperature Sensitivity**

- Do you feel more comfortable in warm or cold weather?
- Are your hands and feet usually warm or cold?

**5. Sweating**

- Do you sweat excessively or very little?
- Is there any specific area where you sweat the most (head, hands, feet)?
- Any noticeable odour in sweat?

### 6. Sexual Health

- Any history of sexual dysfunction, lack of libido, or excessive desire?
- Any past trauma affecting sexual health?

---

### E. Specific Organ-Based Symptoms

1. **Head:** Headaches, dizziness, memory loss, concentration issues.
2. **Eyes:** Vision problems, dry eyes, excessive tearing, photophobia.
3. **Ears:** Hearing issues, ringing, ear infections.
4. **Nose:** Sinus infections, frequent colds, nasal congestion.
5. **Mouth & Throat:** Ulcers, bad breath, sore throat.
6. **Chest & Lungs:** Asthma, breathlessness, cough patterns.
7. **Heart & Circulatory System:** Palpitations, high/low blood pressure.
8. **Stomach & Digestion:** Gas, bloating, acidity, constipation, diarrhea.
9. **Urinary System:** Frequent urination, pain, infections.
10. **Reproductive System:** Menstrual irregularities, pregnancy history.
11. **Musculoskeletal System:** Joint pain, stiffness, back pain.
12. **Skin & Hair:** Dryness, acne, hair fall, eczema.

### F. Modalities & Aggravating/Ameliorating Factors

- What makes your symptoms worse? (Time of day, food, weather, emotions, exertion)
- What relieves your symptoms? (Rest, warmth, cold application, food, sleep)

---

### G. Homoeopathic Constitutional Traits

- Do you have any peculiar habits or mannerisms?
- Any superstitions or unusual fears?
- How do you respond to stress – flight, fight, or freeze?
- Any personal or family history of addiction?

---

### H. Conclusion & Analysis

*A thorough case-taking process not only helps in selecting the most appropriate Homoeopathic remedy but also provides deep insights into the patient's emotional and physical constitution.*

---

## Chapter 18: Psychodynamics of Emotions and Their Role in Disease

### Introduction

Human emotions are deeply tied to health and disease. Anxiety, fear, anger, and sadness are not just psychological states but also influence bodily functions. In homoeopathy, emotional and mental states are considered key factors in the selection of remedies. This chapter explores the psychodynamics of emotions, adaptation mechanisms, and their impact on disease.

---

### 1. Anxiety: The Root Emotion

Anxiety can be considered the **"mother emotion,"** giving rise to:

- **Fear** (linked to the future)
- **Sadness** (linked to loss)
- **Anger** (linked to contradiction or resistance)

**Homoeopathic Perspective**

- **Aconitum Napellus** – Useful for sudden anxiety, fear of death, and restlessness.
- **Argentum Nitricum** – For anticipatory anxiety, impulsiveness, and a sense of urgency.
- **Gelsemium** – Treats performance anxiety, weakness from fear, and trembling.

---

### 2. Adaptation and the Fight-Flight-Freeze Response

When faced with fear or stress, humans adapt using three primary responses:

1. **Flight** → Avoidance or escape from the situation.
2. **Fight** → Facing the challenge head-on.
3. **Freeze** → A state of being stuck or paralyzed.

**Homoeopathic Remedies for Adaptation Reactions**

- **Arsenicum Album** – For individuals prone to avoidance due to anxiety and perfectionism.
- **Nux Vomica** – Helps those who "fight" by being aggressive or overly competitive.
- **Opium** – Useful for cases where a person is emotionally "frozen" due to trauma.

---

### 3. The Energy of Emotions and Disease

Emotions are a form of energy, and when not processed properly, they can manifest as physical symptoms. Stress can be transferred, absorbed, or dissipated, affecting the body's energy balance.

**Key Emotional Energy States**

- **Balanced Emotional Energy** → Leads to adaptability and resilience.
- **Blocked Emotional Energy** → Causes stress, leading to psychosomatic conditions.
- **Excessive Emotional Energy** → Manifests as restlessness, hyperactivity, or even mania.

**Homoeopathic Approach to Emotional Energy Imbalance**

- **Phosphorus** – For individuals who absorb emotions from others, leading to burnout.
- **Calcarea Carbonica** – Helps those who feel overwhelmed by stress and responsibilities.
- **Lachesis** – Useful for intense emotional suppression leading to physical ailments.

## 4. Psychological and Spiritual States

Extreme emotional states can lead to altered states of consciousness:

- **Coma** (complete shutdown)
- **Death** (metaphorical or real, due to energy depletion)
- **Intoxication** (escape via substances)
- **Saintly Intelligence** (higher consciousness and wisdom)

### Homoeopathic Remedies for Psychological States

- **Opium** – For states of unconsciousness or detachment from reality.
- **Cannabis Indica** – Useful for dissociation, altered perceptions, and hallucinations.
- **Aurum Metallicum** – For deep depression and suicidal tendencies.

## 5. Thought, Beliefs, and Stress

- Thoughts and beliefs shape emotional responses.
- Stress is often a result of cognitive dissonance (a conflict between beliefs and reality).
- Chronic stress affects metabolism, electrolyte balance, and circulation, leading to disease.

### Homoeopathic Approach

- **Natrum Muriaticum** – For those who suppress emotions due to rigid beliefs.

- **Ignatia Amara** – Helps with grief, emotional contradictions, and sensitivity.
- **Silicea** – Useful for individuals struggling with self-worth and societal expectations.

---

**Conclusion**

*Understanding the psychodynamics of emotions provides deeper insight into disease formation and treatment. homoeopathy, with its holistic approach, addresses these emotional imbalances, restoring harmony between mind and body.*

---

## Chapter 19:Psychodynamics and Healing: Integrating homoeopathy and Counselling

**Introduction:**

**1.The Interplay of Mind and Body**

Healing is not just about addressing physical symptoms; it requires understanding deep-seated emotional and psychological patterns. The psychodynamic model suggests that unresolved subconscious conflicts manifest as physical ailments. homoeopathy, with its holistic approach, acknowledges this connection, treating not just the disease but the individual as a whole.

**Key Concepts:**

- **The Mind-Body Connection** – How emotions and thoughts influence bodily functions.
- **homoeopathy as Energy Medicine** – How Homoeopathic remedies act beyond the physical level.

- **Vital Force & Healing** – The concept of an energetic force that governs health and disease.

By integrating homoeopathy with psychodynamic counselling, we can uncover hidden mental conflicts and assist the body in healing itself naturally.

---

## 2. Thought, Belief, and Emotional Influence on Health

Every thought and emotion generates a physiological response in the body. Positive emotions promote healing, while prolonged stress and negativity can weaken immunity and contribute to chronic conditions.

**Understanding the Role of Thought and Belief:**

- **Placebo & Nocebo Effect** – How belief alone can heal or harm.
- **Emotional Energy in Cells** – The role of cellular memory in disease patterns.
- **Impact of Childhood Conditioning** – How past experiences create subconscious health scripts.

**Example:** A person who grew up feeling unworthy may develop a pattern of self-neglect, leading to digestive or metabolic issues. A Homoeopathic remedy selected based on their emotional and physical profile can address this at the root level.

---

## 3. Stress as the Root of Disease

Stress is a key factor in most modern illnesses. While short-term stress is beneficial, chronic stress disrupts the body's balance, leading to conditions like hypertension, hormonal imbalances, and autoimmune disorders.

**How Stress Creates Disease:**

- **The Gut-Brain Axis** – Why anxiety can lead to irritable bowel syndrome (IBS).
- **Emotional Suppression & Organ Dysfunction** – How unresolved grief affects lung function, and anger impacts the liver.
- **Chronic Fatigue & Burnout** – How long-term emotional stress results in adrenal exhaustion.

**Real-Life Case:** A patient with chronic migraines may find relief not just through a Homoeopathic remedy but by exploring suppressed frustration or perfectionist tendencies through psychodynamic therapy.

---

**4. Energy, Consciousness, and Healing**

Everything in the universe, including the human body, is composed of energy. Disruptions in energy flow lead to disease, while restoring balance promotes healing. homoeopathy works by stimulating the body's natural healing mechanism.

**Exploring Energy Medicine:**

- **Quantum Physics & Healing** – How thoughts and emotions influence energy fields.
- **The Role of Chakras & Meridians** – Understanding the body's energy pathways.

- **Why homoeopathy Works Energetically** – The law of similar and vibrational healing.

**Example:** A person suffering from chronic allergies may have a deep-seated fear of external threats. A remedy like *Silicea* could help address both their physical and emotional hypersensitivity.

---

### 5. The Psychodynamics of Disease Manifestation

Many diseases can be understood as metaphors for unresolved emotions:

- **Throat issues** → symbolize unexpressed emotions.
- **Back pain** → indicates emotional burdens.
- **Skin conditions** → represent boundary issues or repressed anger.

**How Emotional Conflicts Turn into Physical Symptoms:**

- **Suppression vs. Expression** – Why repressed emotions manifest as chronic conditions.
- **The Body Speaks** – Understanding symptoms as messages from the subconscious.
- **Symbolism of Disease** – Common emotional-physical correlations.

**Example:** A patient experiencing recurrent UTIs may have underlying resentment or unresolved trauma related to relationships. Addressing both the physical symptoms (*Cantharis*, *Staphysagria*) and the emotional pattern through counselling can lead to lasting relief.

---

### 6. Healing the Mind to Heal the Body

True healing involves both physical and emotional transformation. The role of a homoeopath extends beyond prescribing remedies—it involves guiding patients to uncover deeper emotional wounds.

**Approach to Healing:**

1. **Psychodynamic Case Taking** – Identifying emotional themes behind physical symptoms.
2. **Selecting the Right Remedy** – Matching the patient's personality, emotions, and physical symptoms.
3. **Counselling for Awareness** – Helping the patient recognize subconscious patterns.
4. **Lifestyle & Mindfulness Practices** – Supporting the healing journey through meditation, journaling, and healthy routines.

By combining homoeopathy with self-awareness and counselling, patients not only recover from illness but also gain emotional resilience.

---

### 7. Conclusion: The Path to Wholeness

*Health is a dynamic state of balance between the body, mind, and emotions. When we address disease at its deepest level—by understanding and resolving underlying conflicts—we achieve true healing.*

**Final Thoughts:**

- **Prevention is Better than Cure** – How self-awareness can prevent future illnesses.

- **Empowering the Patient** – Teaching individuals to listen to their body's signals.
- **A Holistic Approach to Healing** – Integrating homoeopathy, psychodynamics, and lifestyle changes for complete well-being.

---

## Chapter 20: Psychological Conflict and Disease Manifestation

### Introduction

Psychological conflict is a major contributor to disease, as unresolved inner struggles can manifest as physical ailments. In psychology, conflict arises when a person experiences contradictory desires, beliefs, or emotions, leading to stress and disharmony. From a Homoeopathic perspective, such conflicts disturb the vital force, creating an imbalance that eventually results in disease. This chapter explores the relationship between psychological conflict and disease manifestation, integrating psychodynamic concepts with Homoeopathic understanding.

### 1. Conflict as the Root of Disease

The human mind constantly navigates between desires, societal norms, emotional experiences, and rational thought. When these forces clash, they generate inner conflict, which, if unresolved, creates prolonged stress and energy blockages. Over time, these blockages affect physiological functions, leading to chronic illnesses.

### The Mind-Body Connection

- Emotional suppression or unresolved stress weakens the immune system.

- Chronic stress leads to hormonal imbalances and inflammatory responses.
- The vital force, when disturbed, manifests symptoms as the body's way of signalling distress.

**2. Types of Psychological Conflict and Their Disease Manifestation**

| **Type of Conflict** | **Description** | **Example of Conflict** | **Possible Disease Manifestation** |
|---|---|---|---|
| **Approach-Approach Conflict** | Two equally desirable choices create stress. | Choosing between two dream job offers. | Anxiety disorders, nervous system exhaustion. |
| **Avoidance-Avoidance Conflict** | Two equally undesirable choices cause mental strain. | Staying in a toxic job or facing unemploymen t. | Chronic fatigue, digestive issues, migraines. |
| **Approach-Avoidance Conflict** | A single situation has both positive and negative aspects. | Wanting to start a business but fearing failure. | Gastric ulcers, hypertension, heart disease. |
| **Double Approach-Avoidance Conflict** | Multiple options with both good and bad aspects create extreme stress. | Choosing between career success (but no family time) or family life (but financial instability). | Autoimmune diseases, metabolic disorders. |

### 3. The Role of Thoughts and Beliefs in Disease Creation

- **Rigid beliefs** (e.g., "I must be perfect") create **self-imposed pressure**, leading to conditions like hypertension.
- **Unfulfilled desires** (e.g., emotional repression) cause **energy blockages**, weakening the immune system.
- **Fear-based thinking** (e.g., fear of failure, abandonment) keeps the body in chronic **stress mode**, resulting in hormonal imbalances and chronic diseases.

**Example:** A person suppressing anger due to a belief that expressing anger is wrong may develop **liver disorders**, which homoeopathy often associates with suppressed emotions like anger and resentment.

### 4. Symbolism of Disease as a Reflection of Conflict

Each disease holds a symbolic meaning related to unresolved inner conflict. Some examples include:

- **Asthma** → Fear of expressing oneself or suppressed grief.
- **Skin diseases** → Suppressed emotions or boundary issues.
- **Thyroid disorders** → Conflict between speaking out and staying silent.

### 5. Psychodynamic View: Emotional Repression Leading to Chronic Illness

- Sigmund **Freud's theory**: Repressed emotions resurface as physical symptoms (hysteria, psychosomatic illness).
- Carl **Jung's shadow theory**: Unacknowledged aspects of the self manifest as diseases.
- **Homoeopathic miasms** align with this view:

- **Psora (deep-seated insecurity, fear of lack)** → Skin diseases, anxiety.
- **Sycosis (suppressed emotions, indulgence)** → Tumours, obesity.
- **Syphilis (destructive tendencies, guilt)** → Autoimmune diseases, mental disorders.

### Conclusion: Conflict Resolution as Healing

*Recognizing and resolving inner conflicts helps restore balance to both mind and body. Homoeopathic remedies, by addressing the underlying emotional state, harmonize the disturbed vital force. By integrating* ***psychodynamic counselling with homoeopathy****, practitioners can offer a truly holistic approach to healing.*

---

## Chapter 21:The Psychodynamics of Disease Manifestation – Understanding Emotional Roots and Therapeutic Approaches

---

### Nervous System & Mental Health Disorders

| Physical Symptom / Disorder | Emotional Conflict / Symbolism | Homoeopathic Remedies |
|---|---|---|
| **Headaches / Migraines** | Stress, suppressed anger, excessive responsibility | Belladonna, Nux Vomica, Sanguinaria |
| **Insomnia** | Overthinking, unresolved anxieties, deep fears | Coffea Cruda, Nux Vomica, Passiflora |

| Physical Symptom / Disorder | Emotional Conflict / Symbolism | Homoeopathic Remedies |
|---|---|---|
| **Anxiety disorders** | Overstimulation, fear of the unknown, unresolved trauma | Aconite, Arsenicum Album, Gelsemium |
| **Depression** | Suppressed grief, loss of purpose, emotional exhaustion | Natrum Mur, Aurum Met, Ignatia |
| **OCD (Obsessive-Compulsive Disorder)** | Fear of losing control, suppressed emotions, perfectionism | Syphilinum, Arsenicum Album, Lycopodium |
| **Phobias (irrational fears)** | Deep-seated fear, past traumas resurfacing | Aconitum, Gelsemium, Stramonium |
| **Panic attacks** | Fear of death, lack of security, emotional hypersensitivity | Aconite, Kali Phos, Argentum Nit |
| **PTSD (Post-Traumatic Stress Disorder)** | Unresolved past trauma, deep fear, emotional paralysis | Opium, Stramonium, Arnica |
| **Bipolar disorder** | Emotional instability, unresolved internal conflict | Aurum Met, Anacardium, Ignatia |
| **Schizophrenia** | Fear of reality, fragmented sense of self, detachment | Hyoscyamus, Stramonium, Anacardium |
| **Parkinson's disease** | Fear of losing control, suppressed emotions over time | Zincum Metallicum, Agaricus, Mercurius |

| **Physical Symptom / Disorder** | **Emotional Conflict / Symbolism** | **Homoeopathic Remedies** |
|---|---|---|
| **Alzheimer's / Dementia** | Escaping reality, unresolved past conflicts | Baryta Carb, Anacardium, Alumina |
| **Vertigo / Dizziness** | Inner instability, lack of balance in life | Conium, Gelsemium, Cocculus |
| **Seizures / Epilepsy** | Repressed emotions, inner turmoil, nervous overload | Cicuta, Cuprum Met, Bufo Rana |
| **Multiple Sclerosis (MS)** | Deep frustration, feeling trapped, loss of personal power | Causticum, Plumbum Met, Gelsemium |
| **Neuropathy (nerve pain, tingling, numbness)** | Emotional disconnection, suppressed grief | Hypericum, Phosphorus, Arsenicum Alb |
| **Bell's palsy (facial paralysis)** | Fear of self-expression, sudden emotional shock | Causticum, Aconite, Gelsemium |
| **Tinnitus (ringing in ears)** | Overstimulation, emotional tension, inability to "tune out" stress | Chininum Sulph, Salicylic Acid, Kali Mur |
| **Stroke (post-stroke effects)** | Suppressed anger, feeling powerless, emotional rigidity | Arnica, Lachesis, Nux Vomica |
| **Chronic Fatigue Syndrome (CFS)** | Deep exhaustion, emotional burnout, suppression of desires | Phosphoric Acid, Silicea, Gelsemium |
| **Restless Leg Syndrome (RLS)** | Inner restlessness, inability to relax | Zincum Met, Tarentula, Rhus |

| Physical Symptom / Disorder | Emotional Conflict / Symbolism | Homoeopathic Remedies |
|---|---|---|
| | | Tox |
| **Autism Spectrum Disorder (ASD)** | Sensory overload, deep internal world, difficulty with emotional connection | Carcinosin, Baryta Carb, Agaricus |
| **ADHD (Attention Deficit Hyperactivity Disorder)** | Mental overstimulation, difficulty focusing, hyperactivity | Tuberculinum, Tarentula, Stramonium |
| **Hysteria / Conversion Disorder** | Emotional suppression, internalized trauma, subconscious seeking attention | Ignatia, Stramonium, Moschus |
| **Dissociative Identity Disorder (DID)** | Severe past trauma, fragmentation of identity, emotional protection mechanism | Anacardium, Stramonium, Hyoscyamus |

---

**Digestive System Disorders**

| Condition | Emotional Conflict / Symbolism | Homoeopathic Remedies |
|---|---|---|
| **Acid Reflux / GERD** | Suppressed anger, frustration, inability to express oneself | Nux Vomica, Natrum Mur, Carbo Veg |
| **Indigestion / Dyspepsia** | Anxiety, worry, fear of the future, digestive inefficiency | Lycopodium, Argentum Nitricum, Pulsatilla |
| **Irritable Bowel** | Stress, fear of losing | Nux Vomica, |

| Condition | Emotional Conflict / Symbolism | Homoeopathic Remedies |
|---|---|---|
| **Syndrome (IBS)** | control, unresolved emotional issues | Colocynthis, Chamomilla |
| **Crohn's Disease** | Unresolved grief, feeling of emotional isolation | Calcarea Phosphorica, Bryonia, Sulphur |
| **Ulcerative Colitis** | Anger, frustration, long-held resentment towards others | Aloe Socotrina, Phosphorus, Natrum Sulphuricum |
| **Stomach Ulcers** | Deep-rooted anxiety, chronic stress, lack of emotional release | Argentum Nitricum, Kali Bichromicum, Carbo Veg |
| **Gastritis** | Unexpressed anger, frustration, holding onto hurtful emotions | Nux Vomica, Pulsatilla, Arsenicum Album |
| **Gallstones** | Holding onto bitterness, unprocessed emotions, feeling "stuck" | Chelidonium, Lycopodium, Calcarea Carbonica |
| **Liver Cirrhosis** | Deep resentment, inability to forgive, self-rejection | Carduus Marianus, Phosphorus, Chelidonium |
| **Fatty Liver Disease** | Emotional suppression, unresolved emotional trauma | Taraxacum, Nux Vomica, Lycopodium |
| **Hepatitis** | Repressed anger, frustration, feeling overwhelmed or helpless | Carduus Marianus, Chelidonium, Phosphorus |
| **Pancreatitis** | Emotional overload, unresolved grief, feeling of betrayal | Lycopodium, Arsenicum Album, Phosphorus |

| Condition | Emotional Conflict / Symbolism | Homoeopathic Remedies |
|---|---|---|
| **Constipation** | Emotional blockage, fear of letting go, control issues | Opium, Bryonia, Alumina |
| **Diarrhea** | Fear, anxiety, lack of emotional stability | Argentum Nitricum, Podophyllum, Chamomilla |
| **Malabsorption** | Fear of not being able to "digest" life, emotional insecurity | Lycopodium, Calcarea Carbonica, Carbo Veg |
| **Celiac Disease** | Emotional rigidity, an inability to tolerate life's challenges | Natrum Mur, Calcarea Carbonica, Sulphur |
| **Acute Gastroenteritis** | Anxiety, fear, emotional stress affecting digestion | Arsenicum Album, Ipecacuanha, Veratrum Album |
| **Diverticulitis** | Deep-seated resentment, inability to move forward emotionally | Lycopodium, Colocynthis, Phosphorus |
| **Hemorrhoids** | Suppressed anger, embarrassment, unwillingness to let go | Aesculus Hippocastanum, Hamamelis, Nux Vomica |
| **Fecal Incontinence** | Lack of control, fear of letting go, repressed emotions | Causticum, Opium, Lycopodium |
| **Leaky Gut Syndrome** | Emotional vulnerability, inability to shield oneself emotionally | Natrum Muriaticum, Sulphur, Pulsatilla |
| **Food Allergies / Sensitivities** | Fear of being overwhelmed, feeling | Apis Mellifica, Arsenicum Album, |

| Condition | Emotional Conflict / Symbolism | Homoeopathic Remedies |
|---|---|---|
| | "unsafe" in one's environment | Natrum Mur |
| **Bloating / Flatulence** | Emotional "pressure," difficulty in expressing emotions | Lycopodium, Carbo Veg, Pulsatilla |
| **Chronic Digestive Disorders** | Long-term stress, unresolved emotional conflicts | Nux Vomica, Pulsatilla, Phosphorus |
| **Hiatal Hernia** | Inability to "stomach" emotional conflict, holding on to hurt | Natrum Muriaticum, Carbo Veg, Kali Carbonicum |
| **Gastrointestinal Reflux Disease (GERD)** | Unresolved anger, emotional conflict with life situations | Nux Vomica, Carbo Veg, Phosphorus |
| **Stomach Cancer** | Unresolved anger, frustration, self-rejection, deep emotional hurt | Phosphorus, Calcarea Carbonica, Natrum Mur |
| **Pancreatic Cancer** | Deep emotional trauma, repressed anger, feelings of betrayal | Arsenicum Album, Phosphorus, Lycopodium |
| **Lactose Intolerance** | Anxiety, inability to digest life's experiences, fear of change | Natrum Mur, Sulphur, Lycopodium |
| **Gallbladder Dysfunction** | Emotional repression, fear of change, holding onto old patterns | Chelidonium, Nux Vomica, Lycopodium |
| **SIBO (Small Intestinal Bacterial** | Emotional overload, digestive dysfunction due to stress | Argentum Nitricum, Carbo Veg, Natrum Mur |

| Condition | Emotional Conflict / Symbolism | Homoeopathic Remedies |
|---|---|---|
| **Overgrowth)** | | |
| **Cholecystitis (Gallbladder inflammation)** | Frustration, bitterness, inability to release emotional burdens | Chelidonium, Lycopodium, Phosphorus |
| **Chronic Pancreatitis** | Unresolved grief, emotional betrayal, chronic emotional pain | Phosphorus, Nux Vomica, Lycopodium |
| **Hemorrhagic Gastritis** | Deep emotional wounds, feeling of emotional betrayal or neglect | Nux Vomica, Phosphorus, Carbo Veg |
| **Peptic Ulcer Disease** | Anxiety, fear, emotional suppression, feeling of "injustice" | Argentum Nitricum, Kali Bichromicum, Carbo Veg |
| **Bile Acid Malabsorption** | Emotional suppression, difficulty in "letting go" | Chelidonium, Carbo Veg, Natrum Sulphuricum |
| **Malnutrition** | Emotional neglect, inability to nourish oneself emotionally | Calcarea Phosphorica, Nux Vomica, Lycopodium |
| **Fistulas (Abnormal connections in intestines)** | Unresolved emotional trauma, breaking down of boundaries | Calcarea Phosphorica, Lycopodium, Sulphur |
| **Gastric Bypass Complications** | Fear of change, inability to "digest" life's challenges | Calcarea Carbonica, Nux Vomica, Phosphorus |
| **Ileus (Intestinal Obstruction)** | Repression of emotional expression, fear of moving forward | Bryonia, Nux Vomica, Carbo Veg |

Respiratory System Disorders

| Condition | Emotional Conflict / Symbolism | Homoeopathic Remedies |
|---|---|---|
| **Asthma** | Fear of suffocation, suppressed emotions, childhood trauma | Arsenicum Album, Blatta Orientalis, Sambucus Nigra |
| **Chronic Obstructive Pulmonary Disease (COPD)** | Deep grief, long-standing emotional suppression | Antimonium Tartaricum, Carbo Veg, Kali Carb |
| **Bronchitis (Acute & Chronic)** | Irritation, frustration, difficulty in expressing oneself | Bryonia, Phosphorus, Hepar Sulph |
| **Pneumonia** | Grief, emotional exhaustion, difficulty in "breathing in" life | Phosphorus, Antimonium Tartaricum, Carbo Veg |
| **Pulmonary Fibrosis** | Feeling of being trapped, suppressed sorrow | Silicea, Lycopodium, Kali Carbonicum |
| **Tuberculosis (TB)** | Deep sadness, long-term emotional burden, self-sacrificing nature | Bacillinum, Tuberculinum, Phosphorus |
| **Lung Cancer** | Suppressed grief, unexpressed anger, deep emotional wounds | Phosphorus, Carcinosin, Conium |
| **Pleurisy** | Fear of losing support, feeling emotionally "stabbed" | Bryonia, Kali Carb, Arnica |
| **Sinusitis (Chronic & Acute)** | Irritation with surroundings, blocked emotions | Kali Bichromicum, Pulsatilla, Silicea |

| **Allergic Rhinitis (Hay Fever)** | Sensitivity to environment, suppressed irritation | Sabadilla, Arsenicum Album, Natrum Mur |
|---|---|---|
| **Nasal Polyps** | Emotional congestion, unprocessed grief | Teucrium Marum Verum, Calcarea Carbonica, Sanguinaria |
| **Deviated Nasal Septum** | Feeling of imbalance, distorted self-image | Calcarea Fluorica, Silicea, Thuja |
| **Postnasal Drip** | Unexpressed emotions, repressed sadness | Hydrastis, Kali Bichromicum, Pulsatilla |
| **Sore Throat / Pharyngitis** | Fear of speaking up, resentment, difficulty expressing emotions | Belladonna, Hepar Sulph, Merc Sol |
| **Tonsillitis** | Repressed anger, inability to express emotions | Baryta Carbonica, Belladonna, Hepar Sulph |
| **Laryngitis** | Suppression of voice, fear of being unheard | Causticum, Phosphorus, Argentum Nitricum |
| **Sleep Apnea** | Fear of losing control, suppressed anxiety | Opium, Lachesis, Ammonium Carbonicum |
| **Snoring** | Resentment, unwillingness to let go | Lemna Minor, Opium, Sambucus |
| **Cystic Fibrosis** | Deep-rooted grief, emotional suffocation | Bacillinum, Calcarea Carbonica, Phosphorus |
| **Emphysema** | Feeling stifled, fear of restriction, sadness | Antimonium Tartaricum, Carbo Veg, Kali Carbonicum |

| **Whooping Cough (Pertussis)** | Anxiety, suppressed emotions, fear | Drosera, Cuprum Metallicum, Coccus Cacti |
|---|---|---|
| **Pulmonary Hypertension** | Emotional pressure, fear of failure | Aurum Metallicum, Lachesis, Glonoinum |
| **Pneumothorax (Collapsed Lung)** | Feeling unsupported, emotional collapse | Arnica, Kali Carbonicum, Phosphorus |
| **Lung Abscess** | Internalized resentment, emotional toxicity | Hepar Sulph, Silicea, Kali Bichromicum |
| **Chronic Cough** | Need for attention, unexpressed sadness | Drosera, Rumex, Spongia |
| **Interstitial Lung Disease** | Suppressed grief, emotional rigidity | Silicea, Phosphorus, Kali Carbonicum |
| **Respiratory Distress Syndrome (RDS)** | Fear of survival, feeling unsupported | Antimonium Tartaricum, Carbo Veg, Sambucus |
| **Aspiration Pneumonia** | Emotional choking, difficulty "swallowing" situations | Arsenicum Album, Lachesis, Baptisia |
| **Occupational Lung Diseases** | Long-standing resentment, feeling trapped in work | Silicea, Carbo Veg, Lycopodium |
| **Hiccups (Persistent)** | Suppressed emotions, emotional hiccups in life | Ignatia, Nux Vomica, Hyoscyamus |
| **Vocal Cord Dysfunction** | Fear of expressing oneself, repressed emotions | Argentum Nitricum, Causticum, Phosphorus |
| **Tracheitis** | Suppressed emotions, difficulty in self-expression | Drosera, Kali Bichromicum, Hepar Sulph |

| | | |
|---|---|---|
| **Mediastinitis** | Deep-seated trauma, emotional pressure | Bryonia, Arsenicum Album, Phosphorus |
| **Upper Respiratory Tract Infections (URTI)** | Emotional overload, stress-related immune suppression | Aconite, Belladonna, Ferrum Phos |
| **Lower Respiratory Tract Infections (LRTI)** | Deep-seated fear, repressed sadness | Phosphorus, Antimonium Tartaricum, Kali Carb |
| **Bronchiectasis** | Long-term emotional suppression, inability to let go | Silicea, Kali Carbonicum, Phosphorus |
| **Pulmonary Embolism** | Blocked emotions, suppressed fear of moving forward | Arnica, Lachesis, Hamamelis |
| **Sarcoidosis (Pulmonary)** | Feeling unrecognized, deep emotional wounds | Silicea, Phosphorus, Calcarea Fluorica |
| **COVID-19 Related Lung Complications** | Anxiety, fear, collective trauma | Arsenicum Album, Phosphorus, Bryonia |
| **Epiglottitis** | Fear of losing control, suppression of emotions | Belladonna, Apis Mellifica, Hepar Sulph |

**Cardiovascular System Disorders**

| Condition | **Emotional Conflict / Symbolism** | **Homoeopathic Remedies** |
|---|---|---|
| **Hypertension** | Suppressed anger, | Natrum Mur, |

| Condition | Emotional Conflict / Symbolism | Homoeopathic Remedies |
|---|---|---|
| **(High Blood Pressure)** | inner tension, pressure to perform | Belladonna, Glonoinum |
| **Hypotension (Low Blood Pressure)** | Lack of motivation, feeling powerless, energy depletion | Carbo Veg, China Officinalis, Gelsemium |
| **Atherosclerosis** | Hardening of emotions, fear of change, emotional rigidity | Aurum Met, Plumbum Met, Secale Cornutum |
| **Coronary Artery Disease (CAD)** | Emotional stress, unresolved grief, fear of heartbreak | Digitalis, Cactus Grandiflorus, Naja |
| **Heart Attack (Myocardial Infarction)** | Extreme emotional strain, feeling of being unloved | Crataegus, Arnica, Lachesis |
| **Angina (Chest Pain)** | Suppressed grief, emotional suffocation | Spigelia, Cactus Grandiflorus, Arsenicum Album |
| **Arrhythmia (Irregular Heartbeat)** | Emotional instability, fear of unpredictability | Digitalis, Lachesis, Aurum Met |
| **Atrial Fibrillation (AFib)** | Fear of chaos, inner restlessness | Cactus Grandiflorus, Gelsemium, Naja |
| **Bradycardia (Slow Heart Rate)** | Lack of enthusiasm, slowed emotional response | Digitalis, Gelsemium, Carbo Veg |
| **Tachycardia (Fast Heart Rate)** | Anxiety, panic, feeling overwhelmed | Aconite, Argentum Nitricum, Coffea Cruda |

| Condition | Emotional Conflict / Symbolism | Homoeopathic Remedies |
|---|---|---|
| **Heart Failure (CHF)** | Feeling unsupported, deep exhaustion, lack of emotional energy | Digitalis, Crataegus, Strophanthus |
| **Cardiomyopathy** | Deep sorrow, emotional trauma, lack of joy | Aurum Met, Cactus Grandiflorus, Digitalis |
| **Endocarditis** | Deep-seated resentment, emotional infection | Pyrogenium, Lachesis, Hepar Sulph |
| **Pericarditis** | Emotional armor, fear of emotional vulnerability | Spigelia, Arsenicum Album, Bryonia |
| **Valvular Heart Disease** | Difficulty in giving/receiving love, emotional blockages | Cactus Grandiflorus, Spongia, Lachesis |
| **Mitral Valve Prolapse** | Fear of rejection, inability to open up emotionally | Aurum Met, Lachesis, Strophanthus |
| **Aortic Aneurysm** | Inner explosion, repressed stress, emotional instability | Lachesis, Baryta Mur, Glonoinum |
| **Aortic Dissection** | Emotional breakdown, overwhelming tension | Baryta Mur, Arnica, Glonoinum |
| **Varicose Veins** | Feeling stuck, lack of progress, suppressed frustration | Hamamelis, Pulsatilla, Vipera |
| **Deep Vein Thrombosis (DVT)** | Emotional stagnation, lack of movement in life | Arnica, Hamamelis, Vipera |

| Condition | Emotional Conflict / Symbolism | Homoeopathic Remedies |
|---|---|---|
| **Pulmonary Embolism** | Blocked emotional flow, suppressed fear of moving forward | Lachesis, Hamamelis, Arsenicum Album |
| **Peripheral Artery Disease (PAD)** | Fear of losing independence, emotional withdrawal | Secale Cornutum, Vipera, Baryta Carb |
| **Raynaud's Disease** | Suppressed emotions, fear of exposure, withdrawal | Agaricus, Secale Cornutum, Carbo Veg |
| **Buerger's Disease** | Anger, resentment, self-destructive emotions | Tabacum, Secale Cornutum, Lachesis |
| **Shock (Cardiogenic, Hypovolemic, etc.)** | Sudden emotional trauma, inability to process grief | Aconite, Opium, Camphora |
| **Hypercholesterolemia (High Cholesterol)** | Emotional hoarding, fear of letting go | Aurum Met, Calcarea Carb, Baryta Mur |
| **Anemia (Iron Deficiency, etc.)** | Lack of joy, feeling drained, emotional suppression | Ferrum Phos, China Officinalis, Natrum Mur |
| **Hemophilia** | Fear of life, lack of emotional resilience | Phosphorus, Lachesis, Arnica |
| **Thrombocytopenia (Low Platelet Count)** | Difficulty in healing emotionally, lack of inner security | Carbo Veg, Hamamelis, Phosphorus |
| **Polycythemia Vera (High RBC count)** | Overburdened emotions, holding onto anger | Phosphorus, Sulphur, Arnica |

| Condition | Emotional Conflict / Symbolism | Homoeopathic Remedies |
|---|---|---|
| **Lymphedema** | Holding onto emotional pain, difficulty in processing grief | Apis Mellifica, Conium, Lycopodium |
| **Leukemia (Blood Cancer)** | Deep inner conflict, long-standing emotional wounds | Carcinosin, Phosphorus, Arsenicum Album |
| **Lymphoma (Hodgkin's & Non-Hodgkin's)** | Suppressed emotional trauma, unresolved past issues | Conium, Phytolacca, Kali Ars |
| **Hemorrhoids (Piles)** | Fear of letting go, holding onto past issues | Aesculus, Hamamelis, Nux Vomica |
| **Arteritis (Inflammation of Arteries)** | Suppressed anger, emotional inflammation | Belladonna, Bryonia, Lachesis |
| **Ischemic Heart Disease** | Feeling starved of love, lack of emotional nourishment | Cactus Grandiflorus, Digitalis, Phosphorus |
| **Hypertrophic Cardiomyopathy** | Deep need for recognition, suppressed grief | Aurum Met, Crataegus, Lycopodium |
| **Dilated Cardiomyopathy** | Fear of failure, feeling overwhelmed by life | Digitalis, Strophanthus, Lachesis |
| **Restrictive Cardiomyopathy** | Rigid emotional boundaries, inability to accept love | Cactus Grandiflorus, Aurum Met, Baryta Carb |

| Condition | Emotional Conflict / Symbolism | Homoeopathic Remedies |
|---|---|---|
| **Ventricular Hypertrophy** | Suppressed drive, excessive responsibility | Baryta Carb, Lycopodium, Digitalis |
| **Myocarditis** | Emotional infection, deep inner anger | Belladonna, Pyrogenium, Arsenicum Album |
| **Rheumatic Heart Disease** | Unresolved guilt, childhood trauma | Spigelia, Cactus Grandiflorus, Aurum Met |
| **Takotsubo Cardiomyopathy (Broken Heart Syndrome)** | Extreme heartbreak, sudden emotional shock | Ignatia, Natrum Mur, Phosphoric Acid |
| **Vasculitis** | Internalized anger, resistance to emotional change | Lachesis, Bryonia, Belladonna |
| **Atrial Septal Defect (ASD)** | Emotional gaps, childhood emotional neglect | Calcarea Carb, Baryta Mur, Natrum Mur |
| **Ventricular Septal Defect (VSD)** | Difficulty in balancing emotions, suppressed pain | Aurum Met, Baryta Carb, Phosphorus |
| **Patent Ductus Arteriosus (PDA)** | Emotional attachment issues, fear of growing up | Calcarea Carb, Pulsatilla, Phosphorus |
| **Coarctation of the Aorta** | Emotional restriction, difficulty in self-expression | Baryta Mur, Lachesis, Arnica |
| **Eisenmenger Syndrome** | Suppressed emotions, deep-seated sadness | Lycopodium, Phosphorus, Baryta |

| Condition | Emotional Conflict / Symbolism | Homoeopathic Remedies |
|---|---|---|
| | | Carb |
| **Wolff-Parkinson-White (WPW) Syndrome** | Overstimulation, excessive energy, feeling restless | Phosphorus, Aconite, Argentum Nitricum |
| **Brugada Syndrome** | Fear of the unknown, suppressed anxiety | Aconite, Arsenicum Album, Digitalis |
| **Postural Orthostatic Tachycardia Syndrome (POTS)** | Feeling unstable, difficulty in standing up to life | Gelsemium, Phosphoric Acid, Sepia |
| **Blue Baby Syndrome** | Emotional detachment, lack of nurturing | Carbo Veg, Phosphorus, Lachesis |

---

**Bone Disorders**

| Condition | Emotional Symbolism | Homoeopathic Remedies |
|---|---|---|
| **Osteoporosis** | Deep insecurity, feeling unsupported or fragile in life | Calcarea Phos, Silicea, Symphytum |
| **Osteopenia** | Fear of instability, lack of strong foundation | Calcarea Fluor, Natrum Mur |
| **Osteoarthritis** | Suppressed resentment, rigidity in thinking | Rhus Tox, Bryonia, Causticum |
| **Rheumatoid Arthritis (RA)** | Deep self-criticism, bottled-up anger, fear of vulnerability | Kali Carb, Causticum, Pulsatilla |
| **Gout** | Suppressed aggression, | Colchicum, Ledum, |

| Condition | Emotional Symbolism | Homoeopathic Remedies |
|---|---|---|
| | materialistic stress | Urtica Urens |
| **Paget's Disease of Bone** | Feeling of being reshaped forcefully by life | Silicea, Calcarea Carb, Symphytum |
| **Osteomyelitis (Bone Infection)** | Unresolved trauma, emotional wounding | Hepar Sulph, Merc Sol, Silicea |
| **Bone Fractures** | Feeling broken, lack of support in a crucial area | Symphytum, Arnica, Calcarea Phos |
| **Scoliosis** | Inner conflict between different emotional directions | Calcarea Carb, Silicea, Ruta |
| **Kyphosis (Hunchback)** | Carrying emotional burdens, suppressed self-worth | Natrum Mur, Silicea, Calc Fluor |
| **Lordosis (Swayback)** | Overcompensation, excessive need for approval | Rhus Tox, Kali Carb, Silicea |
| **Spinal Stenosis** | Feeling trapped, restricted movement in life | Rhus Tox, Calcarea Fluor, Hypericum |
| **Osteomalacia** | Lack of emotional resilience, dependency issues | Calcarea Phos, Silicea, Natrum Mur |
| **Bone Tumors** | Suppressed grief, unresolved emotional shock | Carcinosin, Silicea, Conium |
| **Fibrous Dysplasia** | Feeling of deformity, inner self-rejection | Silicea, Calcarea Fluor, Symphytum |
| **Rickets** | Deep need for nurturing, feeling unsupported | Calcarea Phos, Phosphorus, Silicea |

| Condition | Emotional Symbolism | Homoeopathic Remedies |
|---|---|---|
| **Avascular Necrosis** | Fear of losing one's foundation, resistance to change | Arnica, Syphilinum, Silicea |
| **Multiple Myeloma** | Deep-seated resentment, emotional suppression | Carcinosin, Phosphorus, Merc Sol |

---

## Joint Disorders

| Condition | Emotional Conflict / Symbolism | Homoeopathic Remedies |
|---|---|---|
| **Bursitis** | Pent-up irritation, inability to express frustration | Rhus Tox, Belladonna, Arnica |
| **Tendonitis** | Overworking, pressure to perform, stress | Ruta, Rhus Tox, Arnica |
| **Carpal Tunnel Syndrome** | Feeling trapped, excessive strain from repetitive tasks | Hypericum, Causticum, Ruta |
| **Frozen Shoulder** | Holding back emotions, fear of embracing change | Ferrum Met, Rhus Tox, Sanguinaria |
| **Dislocated Joints** | Loss of stability in life, fear of falling apart | Arnica, Symphytum, Rhus Tox |

| Condition | Emotional Conflict / Symbolism | Homoeopathic Remedies |
|---|---|---|
| **TMJ Disorder** | Suppressed anger, inability to express emotions verbally | Ignatia, Belladonna, Causticum |
| **Ankylosing Spondylitis** | Stiffness from suppressed emotions, rigidity in beliefs | Kali Carb, Rhus Tox, Calc Fluor |
| **Polymyalgia Rheumatica** | Emotional exhaustion, lack of flexibility in thinking | Rhus Tox, Gelsemium, Bryonia |
| **Ehlers-Danlos Syndrome** | Feeling stretched beyond limits, fragile emotional state | Calcarea Fluor, Silicea, Ruta |
| **Marfan Syndrome** | Disconnection from the body, self-identity struggles | Phosphorus, Natrum Mur, Silicea |
| **Spondylolisthesis** | Instability, fear of forward movement in life | Rhus Tox, Hypericum, Calc Fluor |
| **Gouty Arthritis** | Suppressed aggression, unresolved anger | Ledum, Colchicum, Urtica Urens |

**Muscle Disorders**

| Condition | Emotional Conflict / Symbolism | Homoeopathic Remedies |
|---|---|---|
| **Muscle Strains & Sprains** | Resistance to change, emotional strain | Arnica, Ruta, Rhus Tox |
| **Fibromyalgia** | Deep-seated emotional trauma, hypersensitivity | Ignatia, Rhus Tox, Phosphoric Acid |
| **Muscular Dystrophy** | Feeling weak, lack of self-expression | Causticum, Gelsemium, Phosphorus |
| **Myositis** | Suppressed rage, feeling burdened | Rhus Tox, Bryonia, Arsenicum |
| **Polymyositis** | Fear of movement, lack of motivation | Causticum, Arnica, Kali Carb |
| **Dermatomyositis** | Feeling exposed, deep-seated vulnerability | Rhus Tox, Natrum Mur, Pulsatilla |
| **Compartment Syndrome** | Feeling trapped, excess internal pressure | Hypericum, Rhus Tox, Arnica |
| **Tennis Elbow** | Frustration from repetitive emotional struggles | Ruta, Rhus Tox, Arnica |
| **Golfer's Elbow** | Internal conflict about self-worth | Rhus Tox, Bellis Perennis |
| **Cramps & Spasms** | Inner tension, unresolved emotional stress | Cuprum Met, Mag Phos, Nux Vomica |

| Condition | Emotional Conflict / Symbolism | Homoeopathic Remedies |
|---|---|---|
| **Restless Leg Syndrome** | Fear of stagnation, deep-seated anxiety | Zincum Met, Tarentula, Agaricus |
| **Myasthenia Gravis** | Weakness from emotional suppression, lack of self-expression | Gelsemium, Causticum, Phosphorus |
| **Rhabdomyolysis** | Emotional overload, inability to release stored emotions | Rhus Tox, Arnica, Arsenicum Alb |
| **Chronic Fatigue Syndrome** | Deep exhaustion, suppressed grief, emotional burnout | Gelsemium, Phosphoric Acid, Silicea |
| **Spinal Muscular Atrophy** | Fear of losing control, powerlessness | Causticum, Gelsemium, Zincum Met |

---

**Spinal & Back Disorders**

| Condition | Emotional Conflict / Symbolism | Homoeopathic Remedies |
|---|---|---|
| **Herniated Disc** | Feeling unsupported, pressure in life | Hypericum, Rhus Tox, Calc Fluor |
| **Sciatica** | Suppressed fear, unresolved emotional stress | Colocynthis, Mag Phos, Bryonia |
| **Lumbago (Lower Back** | Lack of emotional support, carrying | Rhus Tox, Arnica, Kali Carb |

| Condition | Emotional Conflict / Symbolism | Homoeopathic Remedies |
|---|---|---|
| **Pain)** | burdens | |
| **Cervical Spondylosis** | Rigid thought patterns, fear of letting go | Calcarea Carb, Rhus Tox, Kalmia |
| **Whiplash Injury** | Shock, sudden emotional impact | Arnica, Hypericum, Ruta |
| **Tailbone Pain (Coccydynia)** | Feeling unsupported, deep-rooted emotional trauma | Hypericum, Ruta, Nat Mur |
| **Sacroiliitis** | Fear of moving forward in life | Rhus Tox, Kali Carb, Bryonia |
| **Scheuermann's Disease** | Suppressed guilt, carrying the past | Silicea, Nat Mur, Calc Fluor |
| **Spinal Cord Injury (SCI)** | Loss of control, feeling disconnected from life's movement | Hypericum, Arnica, Phosphorus |

---

Thyroid Disorders

| Condition | Emotional Conflict / Symbolism | Homoeopathic Remedies |
|---|---|---|
| **Hypothyroidism** | Suppressed self-expression, feeling unheard or unimportant | Calcarea Carb, Sepia, Natrum Mur |
| **Hyperthyroidism** | Overwhelming | Iodum, Lycopus, |

| Condition | Emotional Conflict / Symbolism | Homoeopathic Remedies |
|---|---|---|
| **(Graves' Disease)** | pressure, inability to slow down | Phosphorus |
| **Hashimoto's Thyroiditis** | Self-directed anger, feeling attacked from within | Thyroidinum, Natrum Mur, Calc Carb |
| **Goiter** | Fear of speaking out, feeling choked emotionally | Spongia, Iodum, Bromium |
| **Thyroid Nodules** | Repressed communication, unspoken emotional pain | Conium, Baryta Carb, Lycopodium |

---

**Diabetes & Blood Sugar Disorders**

| Condition | Emotional Conflict /Symbolism | Homoeopathic Remedies |
|---|---|---|
| **Type 1 Diabetes** | Feeling unsupported, deep fear of abandonment | Phosphorus, Carcinosin, Syzygium |
| **Type 2 Diabetes** | Suppressed joy, emotional sweetness missing in life | Syzygium, Uranium Nit, Lycopodium |
| **Hypoglycemia (Low Blood Sugar)** | Lack of emotional stability, fear of loss | Argentum Nit, Phosphoric Acid, Kali Phos |
| **Insulin Resistance** | Resentment and resistance to change | Syzygium, Thuja, Lycopodium |
| **Gestational** | Fear of nurturing, | Syzygium, Uranium |

| Condition | Emotional Conflict /Symbolism | Homoeopathic Remedies |
|---|---|---|
| **Diabetes** | emotional burden in pregnancy | Nit, Natrum Mur |

## Adrenal Disorders (Stress & Fatigue)

| Condition | Emotional Conflict / Symbolism | Homoeopathic Remedies |
|---|---|---|
| **Adrenal Fatigue** | Chronic stress, feeling overwhelmed and depleted | Gelsemium, Phosphoric Acid, Selenium |
| **Cushing's Syndrome** | Fear of being vulnerable, emotional suppression | Calcarea Carb, Thuja, Natrum Mur |
| **Addison's Disease** | Extreme burnout, loss of personal power | Phosphorus, Arsenicum Alb, Kali Phos |
| **Hyperaldosteronism** | Chronic tension, fear of losing control | Natrum Mur, Kali Carb, Lycopodium |

## Pituitary & Growth Disorders

| Condition | Emotional Conflict / Symbolism | Homoeopathic Remedies |
|---|---|---|
| **Gigantism** | Feeling pressured to be bigger than life, overburdened | Phosphorus, Baryta Carb, Calc Phos |
| **Acromegaly** | Unresolved emotional trauma, feeling forced into a larger role | Baryta Carb, Silicea, Calcarea Carb |
| **Dwarfism (Growth** | Feeling suppressed or stunted emotionally | Baryta Carb, Silicea, Calcarea Phos |

| Condition | Emotional Conflict / Symbolism | Homoeopathic Remedies |
|---|---|---|
| Hormone Deficiency) | | |
| Hyperprolac tinemia | Over-nurturing, excessive emotional dependency | Pulsatilla, Natrum Mur, Phosphorus |

---

**Reproductive Hormonal Disorders**

| Condition | Emotional Conflict / Symbolism | Homoeopathic Remedies |
|---|---|---|
| **Polycystic Ovary Syndrome (PCOS)** | Repressed femininity, fear of self-expression | Apis, Sepia, Pulsatilla |
| **Menopause Symptoms** | Fear of aging, transition resistance | Sepia, Lachesis, Glonoinum |
| **Premenstrual Syndrome (PMS)** | Emotional sensitivity, unresolved stress | Natrum Mur, Sepia, Lachesis |
| **Endometriosis** | Deep-seated emotional pain, self-rejection | Sepia, Lachesis, Thuja |
| **Infertility** | Fear of failure, deep-rooted self-doubt | Natrum Mur, Sepia, Phosphorus |
| **Low Testosterone (Men)** | Feeling powerless, loss of confidence | Agnus Castus, Lycopodium, Selenium |
| **Erectile Dysfunction** | Performance anxiety, fear of inadequacy | Lycopodium, Agnus Castus, Nux Vomica |

---

Kidney Disorders

| Condition | Emotional Conflict / Symbolism | Homoeopathic Remedies |
|---|---|---|
| **Kidney Stones** | Deep-seated resentment, unresolved anger, difficulty letting go | Berberis Vulgaris, Lycopodium, Sarsaparilla |
| **Chronic Kidney Disease (CKD)** | Fear of survival, feeling drained and unsupported | Arsenicum Album, Apis, Lycopodium |
| **Acute Kidney Failure** | Shock, sudden emotional trauma, deep fear | Terebinthina, Apis, Arsenicum Alb |
| **Glomerulonephritis** | Feeling attacked, internalized anger or guilt | Mercurius, Cantharis, Apis |
| **Nephrotic Syndrome** | Overwhelming emotional burden, fear of loss | Apis, Arsenicum Album, Natrum Mur |
| **Polycystic Kidney Disease (PKD)** | Generational trauma, inherited emotional conflict | Lycopodium, Calcarea Carb, Medorrhinum |
| **Hydronephrosis** | Feeling emotionally blocked, resistance to flow in life | Lycopodium, Apis, Terebinthina |
| **Renal Hypertension** | Deep stress, fear of control issues | Glonoinum, Crataegus, Natrum Mur |
| **Renal Colic** | Acute emotional distress, sudden fear or anxiety | Berberis Vulgaris, Colocynthis, Cantharis |

| Condition | Emotional Conflict / Symbolism | Homoeopathic Remedies |
|---|---|---|
| **Medullary Sponge Kidney** | Feeling unable to filter emotions properly | Apis, Terebinthina, Lycopodium |

---

**Bladder Disorders**

| Condition | Emotional Conflict / Symbolism | Homoeopathic Remedies |
|---|---|---|
| **Urinary Tract Infection (UTI)** | Anger in relationships, feeling violated or disrespected | Cantharis, Staphysagria, Apis |
| **Interstitial Cystitis (IC)** | Long-standing emotional pain, frustration in personal life | Cantharis, Equisetum, Natrum Mur |
| **Overactive Bladder** | Fear of losing control, anxiety-driven urgency | Nux Vomica, Causticum, Sepia |
| **Bladder Stones** | Hardening of emotions, holding onto past hurts | Berberis Vulgaris, Sarsaparilla, Lycopodium |
| **Bladder Cancer** | Deep-seated fear, suppressed emotional conflicts | Carcinosin, Thuja, Arsenicum Album |
| **Bladder Atony (Weak Bladder Muscles)** | Loss of willpower, feeling weak emotionally | Causticum, Gelsemium, Staphysagria |
| **Bladder Fistula** | Inability to contain emotions, boundary issues | Silicea, Hepar Sulph, Thuja |

| Condition | Emotional Conflict / Symbolism | Homoeopathic Remedies |
|---|---|---|
| **Neurogenic Bladder** | Loss of control, nervous system overstimulation | Causticum, Gelsemium, Argentum Nit |

---

**Urinary Tract Disorders**

| Condition | Emotional Conflict / Symbolism | Homoeopathic Remedies |
|---|---|---|
| **Urinary Incontinence** | Loss of emotional control, suppressed grief | Causticum, Sepia, Natrum Mur |
| **Difficulty Urinating (Strangury)** | Feeling blocked emotionally, fear of expression | Cantharis, Pareira Brava, Nux Vomica |
| **Nocturnal Enuresis (Bedwetting)** | Childhood trauma, fear of abandonment, insecurity | Cina, Kreosotum, Sepia |
| **Prostatitis** | Suppressed masculinity, emotional tension | Sabal Serrulata, Chimaphila, Lycopodium |
| **Benign Prostatic Hyperplasia (BPH)** | Fear of aging, feeling powerless | Conium, Sabal Serrulata, Baryta Carb |
| **Anuria (No Urine Output)** | Feeling blocked in expressing emotions | Apis, Terebinthina, Cantharis |
| **Polyuria (Excessive Urination)** | Overwhelmed emotions, fear of losing something | Phosphoric Acid, Apis, Natrum Mur |
| **Hematuria** | Deep unresolved | Cantharis, Phosphorus, |

| Condition | Emotional Conflict / Symbolism | Homoeopathic Remedies |
|---|---|---|
| **(Blood in Urine)** | trauma, suppressed grief | Millefolium |
| **Urethritis** | Feeling violated, past emotional wounds | Cantharis, Staphysagria, Mercurius |

---

**Male Reproductive Disorders**

| Condition | Emotional Conflict / Symbolism | Homoeopathic Remedies |
|---|---|---|
| **Erectile Dysfunction (ED)** | Fear of failure, low self-worth, performance anxiety | Agnus Castus, Lycopodium, Caladium |
| **Premature Ejaculation (PE)** | Anxiety, fear of rejection, suppressed guilt | Kali Phos, Nux Vomica, Staphysagria |
| **Low Sperm Count (Oligospermia)** | Fear of inadequacy, deep-seated insecurity | Damiana, Selenium, Acid Phos |
| **Varicocele** | Feeling pressured, burdened responsibilities | Pulsatilla, Hamamelis, Arnica |
| **Prostatitis** | Anger and resentment, suppressed masculinity | Sabal Serrulata, Chimaphila, Lycopodium |
| **Benign Prostatic Hyperplasia (BPH)** | Fear of aging, feeling powerless | Conium, Sabal Serrulata, Baryta Carb |
| **Testicular Pain** | Fear of failure in | Clematis, |

| Condition | Emotional Conflict / Symbolism | Homoeopathic Remedies |
|---|---|---|
| **(Orchialgia)** | relationships, unresolved sexual guilt | Rhododendron, Argentum Nit |
| **Testicular Torsion** | Emotional distress, sudden anxiety | Arnica, Belladonna, Conium |
| **Hydrocele** | Fear of emotional vulnerability, holding onto grief | Rhododendron, Apis, Clematis |
| **Epididymitis** | Unresolved sexual guilt, suppressed resentment | Pulsatilla, Staphysagria, Clematis |
| **Penile Infections (Balanitis)** | Feeling unclean, guilt related to intimacy | Thuja, Mercurius, Nitric Acid |

---

**Female Reproductive Disorders**

| Condition | Emotional Conflict / Symbolism | Homoeopathic Remedies |
|---|---|---|
| **Menstrual Irregularities** | Conflict with femininity, deep-seated fear | Sepia, Pulsatilla, Natrum Mur |
| **Dysmenorrhea (Painful Periods)** | Suppressed anger, rejection of femininity | Mag Phos, Belladonna, Cimicifuga |
| **Amenorrhea (Absent Periods)** | Denial of femininity, fear of womanhood | Sepia, Pulsatilla, Graphites |
| **Menorrhagia (Heavy Bleeding)** | Deep emotional grief, suppressed trauma | Sabina, Trillium, Phosphorus |
| **Polycystic Ovarian** | Fear of losing control, | Thuja, Lachesis, |

| Condition | Emotional Conflict / Symbolism | Homoeopathic Remedies |
|---|---|---|
| **Syndrome (PCOS)** | rejection of self | Pulsatilla |
| **Endometriosis** | Feeling trapped, past unresolved trauma | Sepia, Lachesis, Aurum Met |
| **Fibroids (Uterine Tumors)** | Accumulated emotional pain, suppressed creativity | Calcarea Carb, Sepia, Aurum Mur |
| **Ovarian Cysts** | Deep emotional wounds, suppressed emotions | Thuja, Apis, Lachesis |
| **Vaginitis (Infections, Yeast, Bacterial Vaginosis)** | Fear of intimacy, feeling violated | Kreosotum, Sepia, Merc Sol |
| **Pelvic Inflammatory Disease (PID)** | Sexual guilt, fear of betrayal | Medorrhinum, Merc Sol, Kreosotum |
| **Bartholin's Cyst** | Suppressed sexual energy, unexpressed anger | Silicea, Hepar Sulph, Calc Sulph |
| **Dyspareunia (Painful Intercourse)** | Fear of intimacy, past sexual trauma | Sepia, Kreosotum, Natrum Mur |
| **Vaginismus** | Deep fear of penetration, past trauma | Platina, Ignatia, Sepia |
| **Infertility** | Fear of inadequacy, deep emotional longing | Natrum Mur, Sepia, Calc Phos |
| **Miscarriage / Recurrent Pregnancy Loss** | Deep-seated grief, unresolved trauma | Sabina, Cimicifuga, Secale |
| **Postpartum Depression** | Overwhelming responsibility, fear of | Sepia, Aurum Met, Natrum |

| Condition | Emotional Conflict / Symbolism | Homoeopathic Remedies |
|---|---|---|
| | motherhood | Mur |

## Pregnancy-Related Disorders

| Condition | Emotional Conflict / Symbolism | Homoeopathic Remedies |
|---|---|---|
| **Morning Sickness (Nausea & Vomiting in Pregnancy)** | Fear of new changes, uncertainty in motherhood | Nux Vomica, Sepia, Ipecac |
| **Preeclampsia** | Fear of losing control, deep-seated stress | Belladonna, Lachesis, Veratrum Alb |
| **Gestational Diabetes** | Difficulty receiving love, fear of lack | Syzygium, Uranium Nit, Phosphoric Acid |
| **Preterm Labor** | Feeling unprepared, fear of premature responsibilities | Caulophyllum, Viburnum, Secale |

## Autoimmune Disorders

| Condition | Emotional Conflict / Symbolism | Homoeopathic Remedies |
|---|---|---|
| **Rheumatoid Arthritis (RA)** | Self-attack, deep-seated resentment, difficulty letting go | Causticum, Rhus Tox, Arnica, Kalmia |
| **Lupus (Systemic Lupus Erythematosus - SLE)** | Feeling attacked by life, suppressed self-worth | Sepia, Natrum Mur, Phosphorus |

| Condition | Emotional Conflict / Symbolism | Homoeopathic Remedies |
|---|---|---|
| **Multiple Sclerosis (MS)** | Fear of losing control, feeling stuck, emotional rigidity | Argentum Nit, Causticum, Plumbum Met |
| **Hashimoto's Thyroiditis** | Suppressed self-expression, self-criticism | Iodum, Thyroidinum, Natrum Mur |
| **Graves' Disease (Hyperthyroidism)** | Feeling pressured to perform, unable to slow down | Lycopodium, Nat Mur, Iodum |
| **Psoriasis** | Feeling unprotected, deep-rooted shame, boundary issues | Arsenicum Alb, Graphites, Sulphur |
| **Vitiligo** | Self-rejection, loss of identity, deep emotional trauma | Sepia, Arsenicum Sulph Flavum, Silicea |
| **Type 1 Diabetes** | Rejection of love, feeling unsupported | Phosphoric Acid, Uranium Nit, Syzygium |
| **Sjogren's Syndrome** | Feeling drained, lack of nourishment from life | Natrum Mur, Phosphorus, Lycopodium |
| **Scleroderma** | Emotional rigidity, fear of vulnerability | Silicea, Fluoric Acid, Causticum |
| **Myasthenia Gravis** | Fear of responsibility, feeling powerless | Gelsemium, Argentum Nit, Conium |
| **Autoimmune Hepatitis** | Suppressed anger, difficulty processing emotions | Chelidonium, Lycopodium, Nux Vomica |
| **Celiac Disease** | Rejection of | Natrum Mur, |

| Condition | Emotional Conflict / Symbolism | Homoeopathic Remedies |
|---|---|---|
| | nourishment, deep sensitivity to criticism | Silicea, Lycopodium |
| **Alopecia Areata** | Fear of loss, identity crisis, unresolved grief | Phosphorus, Lycopodium, Sepia |

## Chronic Immune Deficiencies & Infections

| Condition | Emotional Conflict / Symbolism | Homoeopathic Remedies |
|---|---|---|
| **Chronic Fatigue Syndrome (CFS)** | Feeling overwhelmed, emotional burnout, lack of support | Gelsemium, Phosphoric Acid, Arsenicum Alb |
| **HIV/AIDS** | Deep-seated feelings of guilt, rejection, loss of self-worth | Carcinosin, Natrum Mur, Syphilinum |
| **Tuberculosis (TB)** | Suppressed grief, longing for care and support | Tuberculinum, Phosphorus, Silicea |
| **Frequent Colds & Flu** | Feeling emotionally drained, needing rest | Arsenicum Alb, Gelsemium, Aconite |
| **Recurrent Infections** | Fear of being weak, subconscious self-sabotage | Echinacea, Silicea, Hepar Sulph |
| **Sepsis (Blood Infection)** | Deep internal conflict, suppressed emotional pain | Pyrogenium, Lachesis, Baptisia |

Lymphatic System Disorders

| Condition | Emotional Conflict / Symbolism | Homoeopathic Remedies |
|---|---|---|
| **Lymphadenopathy (Swollen Lymph Nodes)** | Fear of exposure, emotional overload | Conium, Merc Sol, Calcarea Carb |
| **Lymphedema** | Holding onto past emotions, suppressed grief | Apis, Calc Fluor, Pulsatilla |
| **Lymphoma (Hodgkin's & Non-Hodgkin's)** | Deep-seated self-rejection, loss of joy | Carcinosin, Arsenicum Alb, Phosphorus |
| **Mononucleosis (Glandular Fever)** | Overburdened with responsibility, exhaustion | Kali Phos, Gelsemium, Natrum Mur |

---

Skin Disorders

| Condition | Emotional Conflict / Symbolism | Homoeopathic Remedies |
|---|---|---|
| **Acne** | Feeling unworthy, self-criticism, suppressed anger | Hepar Sulph, Silicea, Kali Bromatum |
| **Eczema (Atopic Dermatitis)** | Deep sensitivity, suppressed emotions, feeling unsafe | Graphites, Sulphur, Mezereum |
| **Psoriasis** | Feeling unprotected, deep-rooted shame, boundary issues | Arsenicum Alb, Graphites, Sepia |
| **Hives** | Anxiety, fear of | Apis, Natrum Mur, Rhus |

| Condition | Emotional Conflict / Symbolism | Homoeopathic Remedies |
|---|---|---|
| **(Urticaria)** | confrontation, hypersensitivity | Tox |
| **Vitiligo** | Self-rejection, loss of identity, deep emotional trauma | Sepia, Arsenicum Sulph Flavum, Silicea |
| **Rosacea** | Suppressed embarrassment, fear of judgment, self-consciousness | Belladonna, Carbo Veg, Pulsatilla |
| **Fungal Infections (Ringworm, Athlete's Foot, etc.)** | Feeling contaminated, lack of personal boundaries | Sepia, Silicea, Thuja |
| **Boils & Abscesses** | Suppressed anger, repressed emotions | Hepar Sulph, Silicea, Myristica |
| **Keloids & Scars** | Holding onto past emotional wounds | Fluoric Acid, Silicea, Graphites |
| **Hyperpigmentation / Melasma** | Fear of being seen, emotional trauma | Sepia, Thuja, Lycopodium |
| **Ichthyosis (Excessive Dry Skin)** | Deep loneliness, feeling unlovable | Arsenicum Alb, Petroleum, Sulphur |

### Hair Disorders

| Condition | Emotional Conflict / Symbolism | Homoeopathic Remedies |
|---|---|---|
| **Alopecia (Hair Loss, Baldness)** | Fear of loss, identity crisis, unresolved grief | Phosphorus, Lycopodium, Sepia |
| **Premature Graying of Hair** | Stress, emotional exhaustion, fear of aging | Phosphoric Acid, Lycopodium, Nat Mur |
| **Dandruff (Scalp Flaking)** | Anxiety, internal conflict, emotional stress | Thuja, Graphites, Kali Sulph |
| **Seborrheic Dermatitis (Scalp Eczema)** | Emotional overwhelm, inner turmoil | Arsenicum Album, Mezereum, Sulphur |
| **Trichotillomania (Hair Pulling Disorder)** | Compulsive need for control, anxiety | Nat Mur, Arsenicum Alb, Nux Vomica |

---

### Nail Disorders

| Condition | Emotional Conflict / Symbolism | Homoeopathic Remedies |
|---|---|---|
| **Brittle Nails** | Feeling weak, insecurity, self-doubt | Silicea, Calcarea Fluor, Nat Mur |
| **White Spots on Nails (Leukonychia)** | Unexpressed emotions, perfectionism | Silicea, Thuja, Natrum Carb |

| Condition | Emotional Conflict / Symbolism | Homoeopathic Remedies |
|---|---|---|
| **Ingrown Nails** | Feeling trapped, suppressed resentment | Magnetis Polus Australis, Hepar Sulph |
| **Fungal Nail Infections** | Fear of contamination, boundary issues | Silicea, Graphites, Thuja |
| **Clubbing of Nails** | Chronic emotional stress, deep-seated sadness | Arsenicum Alb, Carbo Veg, Antimonium Crud |

## Eye Disorders

| Condition | Emotional Conflict / Symbolism | Homoeopathic Remedies |
|---|---|---|
| **Myopia (Nearsightedness)** | Fear of the future, avoidance of what lies ahead | Phosphorus, Silicea, Ruta |
| **Hyperopia (Farsightedness)** | Difficulty focusing on the present, fear of missing out | Calcarea Carb, Natrum Mur, Lycopodium |
| **Astigmatism** | Distorted perception of reality, inner conflict | Argentum Nit, Physostigma, Gelsemium |
| **Cataracts** | Fear of seeing the truth, emotional clouding | Causticum, Silicea, Natrum Sulph |
| **Glaucoma** | Pressure from unexpressed emotions, holding | Phosphorus, Osmium, Belladonna |

| Condition | Emotional Conflict / Symbolism | Homoeopathic Remedies |
|---|---|---|
| | onto the past | |
| **Macular Degeneration** | Fear of losing independence, grief over aging | Phosphoric Acid, Lycopodium, Aurum Met |
| **Dry Eyes** | Emotional dryness, feeling unfulfilled | Pulsatilla, Euphrasia, Alumina |
| **Conjunctivitis (Pink Eye)** | Suppressed anger, unwillingness to see a situation clearly | Euphrasia, Argentum Nit, Belladonna |
| **Eye Twitching (Blepharospasm)** | Suppressed nervousness, stress overload | Agaricus, Zincum Met, Gelsemium |
| **Strabismus (Crossed Eyes)** | Conflict between logic and emotions, difficulty in decision-making | Cicuta, Gelsemium, Physostigma |

## Ear Disorders

| Condition | Emotional Conflict / Symbolism | Homoeopathic Remedies |
|---|---|---|
| **Hearing Loss (Partial or Complete)** | Avoidance of hearing unpleasant truths, emotional withdrawal | Chenopodium, Phosphorus, Calcarea Fluor |
| **Tinnitus (Ringing in the Ears)** | Overload of external noise, difficulty processing | Salicylic Acid, Natrum Salicylicum, Chininum Sulph |

| Condition | Emotional Conflict / Symbolism | Homoeopathic Remedies |
|---|---|---|
| | emotions | |
| **Ear Infections (Otitis Media)** | Anger, frustration, not wanting to hear conflicts | Chamomilla, Pulsatilla, Belladonna |
| **Meniere's Disease (Vertigo + Tinnitus + Hearing Loss)** | Inner turmoil, feeling emotionally off-balance | Gelsemium, Conium, Chininum Sulph |
| **Vertigo (Dizziness)** | Loss of control, emotional instability | Cocculus, Bryonia, Conium |
| **Hyperacusis (Sensitivity to Sound)** | Emotional hypersensitivity, fear of confrontation | Phosphorus, Nux Vomica, Theridion |
| **Barotrauma (Ear Pressure Changes)** | Fear of external pressure, resistance to change | Arnica, Carbo Veg, Belladonna |

## Nose Disorders

| Condition | Emotional Conflict / Symbolism | Homoeopathic Remedies |
|---|---|---|
| **Sinusitis (Chronic & Acute)** | Suppressed grief, unresolved emotional congestion | Kali Bich, Silicea, Pulsatilla |
| **Nasal Polyps** | Fear of confrontation, difficulty expressing emotions | Teucrium, Calcarea Carb, Thuja |
| **Allergic** | Feeling invaded by | Sabadilla, Arsenicum |

| Condition | Emotional Conflict / Symbolism | Homoeopathic Remedies |
|---|---|---|
| **Rhinitis (Hay Fever)** | external influences, emotional hypersensitivity | Album, Allium Cepa |
| **Postnasal Drip** | Holding back emotions, unexpressed sadness | Kali Sulph, Hydrastis, Natrum Mur |
| **Deviated Nasal Septum** | Conflict between personal and external expectations | Silicea, Calc Fluor, Thuja |
| **Loss of Smell (Anosmia)** | Fear of experiencing new situations, emotional detachment | Pulsatilla, Zincum Met, Natrum Mur |

## Tongue & Taste Disorders

| Condition | Emotional Conflict / Symbolism | Homoeopathic Remedies |
|---|---|---|
| **Glossitis (Tongue Inflammatio n)** | Difficulty expressing emotions, suppressed anger | Nitric Acid, Merc Sol, Arsenicum Alb |
| **Burning Mouth Syndrome** | Lingering emotional pain, unresolved anger | Arsenicum Alb, Phosphorus, Natrum Mur |
| **Loss of Taste (Ageusia)** | Loss of joy, feeling disconnected from experiences | Zincum Met, Pulsatilla, Natrum Mur |
| **Geographic Tongue** | Fear of change, internal inconsistency | Taraxacum, Natrum Mur, Merc Sol |
| **Thrush (Oral Candidiasis)** | Feeling suppressed, difficulty asserting oneself | Borax, Merc Sol, Sulphur |

# Chapter 22: Expression of Emotion and Mind – How to Identify It

## 1. Introduction

The human mind and emotions are deeply interconnected, and their expression plays a crucial role in understanding an individual's psychological state. In homoeopathy, accurate observation of a patient's emotional and mental expressions is vital for case analysis and remedy selection.

This chapter explores:

- The different ways emotions manifest
- Their psychological significance
- How they correlate with Homoeopathic remedies

---

## 2. Understanding Emotional Expression

Emotions can be communicated **verbally and non-verbally**. While spoken words provide direct insight, non-verbal expressions such as **facial movements, posture, and tone of voice** often reveal hidden emotions that the patient may not consciously express. Recognizing these expressions allows homoeopaths to access deeper layers of a patient's psychological state.

### 2.1 Verbal vs. Non-Verbal Expression

- **Verbal Expression** – Direct communication of emotions through speech
- **Non-Verbal Expression** – Unconscious display of emotions through body language, facial expressions, tone, and physiological changes

## 3. Types of Emotional Expressions

### 3.1 Facial Expressions

Facial expressions are among the most powerful indicators of emotions. They often reveal underlying mental states, even when a person attempts to conceal them.

| Emotion | Facial Indicators |
|---|---|
| **Joy** | Smiling, relaxed facial muscles, bright eyes |
| **Sadness** | Drooping eyelids, downturned lips, watery eyes |
| **Anger** | Furrowed brows, tightened jaw, piercing gaze |
| **Fear** | Widened eyes, tense facial muscles, raised eyebrows |
| **Disgust** | Wrinkled nose, curled lips |
| **Surprise** | Raised eyebrows, wide-open eyes, open mouth |

### 3.2 Body Language

Body posture and movements provide valuable clues about emotional states.

- **Open posture** → Confidence, receptivity (e.g., arms relaxed, upright posture)
- **Closed posture** → Defensiveness, insecurity (e.g., crossed arms, slouched shoulders)
- **Fidgeting** → Nervousness, anxiety (e.g., tapping fingers, shifting weight)
- **Avoidance behaviours** → Discomfort or fear (e.g., lack of eye contact, turning away)

### 3.3 Speech Patterns

Tone, pitch, and speech rate often change based on emotional states.

- **Slow, soft voice** → Depression, grief
- **Rapid, high-pitched speech** → Anxiety, excitement
- **Monotone speech** → Apathy, emotional suppression
- **Hesitant speech** → Fear, uncertainty

### 3.4 Physiological Responses

Emotional expression is also reflected in physiological changes:

- **Sweating** → Anxiety, nervousness
- **Pupil dilation** → Interest, attraction, fear
- **Muscle tension** → Stress, anger
- **Rapid breathing** → Panic, excitement

### 3.5 Behavioural Expressions

- **Repetitive habits** → Nail-biting (anxiety), hair twirling (nervousness)
- **Self-isolation** → Depression, withdrawal
- **Explosive reactions** → Unprocessed anger or frustration

---

## 4. Psychological and Homoeopathic Correlations

Each emotional expression can be mapped to specific Homoeopathic remedies:

| Emotional Expression | Homoeopathic Remedy |
| --- | --- |
| **Suppressed grief, avoids consolation** | Natrum Muriaticum |

| Emotional Expression | Homoeopathic Remedy |
|---|---|
| **Frequent sighing, changeable moods** | Ignatia Amara |
| **Deep sadness, suicidal tendencies** | Aurum Metallicum |
| **Weeping easily, need for reassurance** | Pulsatilla |
| **Talkative, intense emotions** | Lachesis |
| **Irritability, impatience** | Nux Vomica |
| **Suppressed anger, resentment** | Staphysagria |

---

## 5. Recognizing Suppressed and Masked Emotions

### 5.1 Conscious Suppression vs. Subconscious Repression

- **Suppressed emotions** → Actively hidden due to societal or personal reasons
- **Repressed emotions** → Buried in the subconscious, often manifesting in physical symptoms

### 5.2 Detecting Hidden Emotions

- Contradictions between speech and body language
- Inconsistent facial expressions
- Sudden changes in voice tone or pace
- Physical complaints without medical explanation

---

## 6. Case Examples

### 6.1 Case of Suppressed Grief (Natrum Muriaticum)

A 40-year-old woman presented with **chronic migraines and insomnia**. Upon questioning, she revealed losing her mother five years ago but insisted she had "moved on." However, her body language showed **tense shoulders and avoidance of eye contact** when discussing her loss. Tears welled up when she was asked about childhood memories. **Natrum Muriaticum** helped her process her grief, and her migraines gradually subsided.

### 6.2 Case of Uncontrolled Anger (Staphysagria)

A 28-year-old man experienced **recurrent skin eruptions** after conflicts at work. He denied being angry but **clenched his jaw and fists** when discussing his workplace issues. After prescribing **Staphysagria**, his emotional suppression lifted, and his skin condition improved.

### 6.3 Case of Anxiety and Nervous Behavior (Argentum Nitricum)

A student with **severe exam anxiety** displayed **rapid speech, excessive hand movements, and a habit of tapping his foot**. He described frequent urges to escape stressful situations. **Argentum Nitricum** helped him regain composure, and his physical restlessness reduced.

### 6.4 Case of Over-Sensitivity to Criticism (Lachesis)

A middle-aged woman became **defensive and spoke excessively** when questioned about her emotions. She often interrupted, contradicting herself, and was highly expressive. **Lachesis** helped her gain self-awareness and regulate her speech patterns.

---

### 7. Practical Techniques for Identifying Emotional Expression

- **Observational techniques** → Careful study of micro-expressions
- **Guided questioning** → Open-ended questions to encourage expression
- **Empathetic mirroring** → Reflecting back emotions to gain clarity
- **Role-playing** → Encouraging patients to express hidden emotions in a safe environment
- **Journaling** → Asking patients to write down thoughts to analyze their emotional patterns

---

### 8. Conclusion

*Understanding* ***emotional expression*** *is key to accurate Homoeopathic case-taking. By integrating* ***observational skills, psychological insights, and Homoeopathic principles****, practitioners can uncover hidden emotional states and select remedies that address both the* ***mental and physical aspects*** *of disease.*

*Mastering this skill enhances treatment outcomes and* ***deepens the patient-practitioner relationship****.*

---

## Chapter 23:The Unspoken Language of Toddlers and Children: Understanding Non-Verbal Cues

In young children and toddlers, **verbal communication is often limited**, making **non-verbal cues essential** in understanding their emotional and physical states. The **unspoken language** in this age group may be subtle but provides valuable insights into their **needs, anxieties, and overall well-being**.

---

1. **Body Language and Gestures**

- **Clinginess or Attachment** → Toddlers may exhibit distress by **holding onto a parent or caregiver**, seeking comfort through **physical closeness**, or refusing to let go. This could indicate **fear, insecurity, or emotional discomfort**.
- **Throwing Objects or Pushing** → Aggressive actions like throwing toys or pushing others may indicate **frustration, anger, or difficulty expressing emotions verbally**.
- **Fidgeting and Restlessness** → Constant movement, pacing, or difficulty sitting still may signal **anxiety, discomfort, or a need for attention**.
- **Withdrawal or Hiding** → If a child withdraws or hides behind a parent, it may reflect **fear, anxiety, or emotional distress**, possibly linked to a **traumatic event or separation anxiety**.

---

2. **Facial Expressions**

- **Furrowed Brows or Pouting** → A child who furrows their brows or pouts may be expressing **confusion, discomfort, or dissatisfaction**, often associated with frustration.
- **Tears Without an Obvious Cause** → Crying without an apparent reason can indicate **emotional discomfort**, such

as **fear, loneliness, or distress due to a change in routine or environment.**

---

### 3. Tone of Voice and Crying

- **Whining or Whimpering** → A high-pitched or constant whine may indicate a **need for reassurance, attention, or comfort**. It could also signal **physical discomfort, such as pain or hunger.**
- **Crying with Varying Intensity** →
    - **Sudden, loud crying** → May indicate **a traumatic event or immediate distress.**
    - **Low, persistent crying** → Could reflect **sadness, loneliness, or a feeling of abandonment.**

---

### 4. Sleep Patterns

- **Difficulty Falling Asleep or Frequent Night Wakings** → May indicate **emotional distress, fears, or even unresolved trauma.**
- **Clinginess Before Bedtime** → If a child suddenly becomes **clingy or afraid to sleep alone**, it may be due to **separation anxiety or fear of being alone.**

---

### 5. Behavioural Changes

- **Regression in Behaviour** → A child suddenly returning to **previous behaviours** (e.g., thumb-sucking, bedwetting) can signal **stress, anxiety, or an emotional setback** due to environmental or routine changes.

- **Overactive or Underactive Behaviour →**
    - **Hyperactivity** may indicate **excitement or overstimulation.**
    - **Lethargy or withdrawal** may indicate **sadness, depression, or emotional exhaustion.**

---

### 6. Importance of Recognizing Non-Verbal Cues

Understanding these non-verbal signs helps **parents and healthcare practitioners** address a child's emotional and physical needs more effectively. Since **non-verbal communication is often the first and most telling way** to understand what a child may be going through, careful **observation and interpretation** are crucial in both diagnosis and treatment.

*By being attuned to these silent signals, Homoeopathic practitioners can* ***better assess emotional imbalances*** *and choose the* ***appropriate remedies*** *to restore harmony in young patients.*

---

## Chapter 24:Rubrics for Emotional and Gesture Connections

Understanding the connection between **emotions and physical gestures** is essential in Homoeopathic case-taking. Non-verbal cues such as **posture, facial expressions, and body movements** offer significant insight into a patient's emotional state. The following rubrics help correlate **gestures with emotional expressions**, aiding in precise remedy selection.

1. **Anger, Irritability, and Gestures**

- **Expression of Anger:** Clenched fists, tight jaw, furrowed brows, sudden outbursts of irritability, punching, or kicking.
- **Rubric:** *Anger, violent, indignation, gestures expressive of*
- **Examples of Remedies:** *Nux Vomica, Staphysagria*

2. **Sadness and Gestures**

- **Expression of Sadness:** Drooping posture, lack of eye contact, sitting with shoulders hunched, sighing, or covering face.
- **Rubric:** *Grief, silent, crying*
- **Examples of Remedies:** *Natrum Muriaticum, Ignatia Amara*

3. **Fear and Gestures**

- **Expression of Fear:** Shivering, wide eyes, clenched body, fidgeting, or avoiding eye contact.
- **Rubric:** *Fear, anxiety, restlessness*
- **Examples of Remedies:** *Argentum Nitricum, Aconite, Gelsemium*

4. Joy and Gestures

- **Expression of Joy:** Smiling, eyes sparkling, relaxed posture, open body language, light movements, or spontaneous laughter.
- **Rubric:** *Joy, happiness, lively*
- **Examples of Remedies:** *Phosphorus, Sepia*

---

5. Anxiety and Gestures

- **Expression of Anxiety:** Fidgeting, rapid speech, nail-biting, pacing, or wringing of hands.
- **Rubric:** *Anxiety, general*
- **Examples of Remedies:** *Argentum Nitricum, Kali Phos, Lycopodium*

---

6. Suppression of Emotions

- **Expression of Emotional Suppression:** Holding back tears, controlling facial expressions, maintaining a stiff posture, or masking true emotions behind a forced smile.
- **Rubric:** *Suppression of emotions*
- **Examples of Remedies:** *Natrum Muriaticum, Pulsatilla*

---

7. Excitement and Gestures

- **Expression of Excitement:** Rapid speech, fidgeting, energetic movements, quick gestures, or restless pacing.

- **Rubric:** *Excitement, restlessness, enthusiasm*
- **Examples of Remedies:** *Coffea Cruda, Chamomilla*

---

**8. Nervousness and Gestures**

- **Expression of Nervousness:** Fidgeting, shifting eyes, biting lips, tapping feet, or wringing hands.
- **Rubric:** *Nervousness, general*
- **Examples of Remedies:** *Argentum Nitricum, Pulsatilla*

---

**9. Indifference and Gestures**

- **Expression of Indifference:** Slumped posture, lack of expression, monotone voice, or lack of movement.
- **Rubric:** *Apathy, indifference, carelessness*
- **Examples of Remedies:** *Calcarea Carbonica, Phosphoric Acid*

---

**10. Confusion and Gestures**

- **Expression of Confusion:** Furrowed brows, head tilting, stuttering, shaking head in disbelief, or blank stares.
- **Rubric:** *Confusion, mental*
- **Examples of Remedies:** *Anacardium, Lac Caninum*

---

### Conclusion

*These rubrics offer* ***a deeper understanding of how physical gestures reflect emotional and mental states****, providing valuable clues in Homoeopathic case analysis. By observing* ***both internal emotional states and external behavioural expressions****, practitioners can select remedies with greater accuracy, ensuring a* ***holistic approach*** *to treatment.*

---

## Chapter 25: Consultation – How to Counsel, Consult, Open, and Close a Case

### 1. Introduction

In homoeopathy, consultation is more than just gathering symptoms; it is about:

- **Building rapport** with the patient.
- **Understanding their complete story**—both physical and emotional.
- **Interpreting verbal and non-verbal cues** to select the most appropriate remedy.

A well-structured consultation **lays the foundation for accurate remedy selection** and supports the patient's healing journey. This chapter covers:

- The art of **opening a case** to establish trust.
- **Effective case-taking techniques** that capture mental, emotional, and physical aspects.
- **Counselling strategies** to support the patient emotionally.
- **Closing a case** with clear guidance on follow-ups and treatment expectations.

---

## 2. Opening a Case: Creating a Comfortable Space

### A. Establishing Rapport

The **first few moments** of a consultation shape the entire process. Patients must feel **heard, respected, and emotionally safe**.

- **Eye contact and body language:** Maintain a welcoming posture and steady yet gentle eye contact.
- **Active listening:** Allow the patient to express freely, without unnecessary interruptions.
- **Empathy and compassion:** Acknowledge their suffering without judgment.

> *Example Statement:*
> "I understand this has been a difficult time for you.
> Feel free to share whatever is on your mind."

### B. Setting the Tone for the Consultation

- Ensure **a calm and inviting atmosphere**.
- Let the patient know that this is a **confidential, open space** where they can discuss anything freely.
- Provide **assurance and emotional safety** to encourage honest communication.

---

## 3. Gathering Case Information

### A. Structure of Case-Taking

A homoeopath must explore **a wide range of information** in a structured manner:

◈ **Mental Symptoms** – Ask about emotional well-being, thought patterns, and stress levels.

- *Example Question:* "How have you been feeling emotionally in the past few weeks?"

◈ **Physical Symptoms** – Document pain, sleep disturbances, appetite changes, and general health.

- *Example Question:* "Have you noticed any changes in your energy levels or digestion?"

◈ **Patient History** – Explore personal and family health history, as emotional or psychological conditions often correlate with physical symptoms.

**B. Observational Skills**

Verbal responses are important, but **non-verbal cues** can be equally revealing:

- **Body Language:** Does the patient seem restless or withdrawn?
- **Facial Expressions:** Do they show emotional suppression or tension?
- **Voice Tone & Speed:** Do they speak rapidly (anxiety) or slowly (depression)?

---

**4. Counselling During the Consultation**

homoeopathy involves **listening and providing gentle guidance**. A homoeopath must create an environment where the patient feels:

1. **Heard** – Their emotions are acknowledged.
2. **Understood** – Their experiences are validated.

3. **Supported** – They feel reassured during their healing process.

### A. Active Listening and Reflection

Reflecting on the patient's emotions encourages them to share more.

> *Example Reflection:*
> "It seems like you're feeling overwhelmed by your current situation."

### B. Managing Sensitive Topics

- Be patient and allow **natural progression** in case-taking.
- Avoid forcing the patient to discuss trauma unless they are **ready to share.**

### C. Emotional Support

- Recognize distress and respond appropriately.
- A simple statement like **"I can see this is difficult for you"** fosters trust.

---

## 5. Analyzing and Connecting Symptoms

### A. Identifying Key Symptoms

1) **Primary Complaint** – What is the main reason for the consultation?

2) **Secondary Symptoms** – How do they relate to the main complaint?

### B. Pattern Recognition

- Are there **recurring emotional or physical patterns**?

- Do certain symptoms **worsen under stress** or **during specific times of the day**?

**C. Remedy Selection**

- Select remedies based on the **totality of symptoms** (mental, emotional, and physical).
- Ensure that the remedy addresses the **mind-body connection**, a core principle in homoeopathy.

---

**6. Closing the Case: Guidance and Follow-up**

**A. Explaining the Treatment Plan**

- **Set clear expectations** – Healing takes time; results vary per individual.
- **Explain the remedy's role** – How it works holistically on the patient's condition.
  ✔ **Dosage & Instructions** – Specify the correct way to take the remedy.

*Example Statement:*
"You may notice subtle changes in your mood or energy before physical symptoms improve."

**B. Managing the Follow-Up Process**

1. **Schedule follow-ups** – Regular assessments help track progress.
2. **Modify treatment if necessary** – Adjust remedies based on symptom evolution.

**C. Closing Remarks**

Offer reassurance and reinforce that **continued care is essential**.

*Example Encouragement:*
"This is a journey, and I am here to support you throughout the process."

---

## 7. Case Studies and Practical Insights

### Case 1: Anxiety-Linked Digestive Issues

**Patient:** 32-year-old woman with digestive complaints.
**Background:** High stress from a demanding job and recent breakup.
**Symptoms:** Rapid speech, high-pitched voice, bloating, nausea, insecurity, and fear of failure.
**Remedy:** *Argentum Nitricum* (for anxiety-induced digestive issues).
**Outcome:** Significant improvement in symptoms after the first dose.

---

### Case 2: Suppressed Anger and Headaches

**Patient:** 45-year-old man with chronic headaches.
**Background:** Tension following a workplace conflict.
**Symptoms:** Appears calm but with tense body language and avoidance of eye contact.
**Remedy:** *Nux Vomica* (for suppressed anger and associated physical symptoms).
**Outcome:** Headaches resolved within weeks, patient felt emotionally lighter.

---

## 8. Conclusion

Effective Homoeopathic consultation is **both an art and a science**. A skilled homoeopath must:

- **Establish trust and rapport** with the patient.

- **Observe, listen, and interpret** both spoken and unspoken cues.
- **Analyze symptoms holistically** to ensure accurate remedy selection.
- **Provide emotional support and clear guidance** throughout treatment.

*A structured yet* ***compassionate approach*** *enhances the healing experience and ensures long-term success in Homoeopathic treatment.*

---

## Chapter 26: Case Studies – Integrating Psychodynamics and homoeopathy

### 1. Introduction

This chapter presents real-world case studies demonstrating the integration of homoeopathy and psychodynamics in treating various conditions. Each case highlights how underlying emotional conflicts manifest as physical ailments and how Homoeopathic remedies facilitate healing by addressing both mind and body.

### 2. Case Studies

#### Case 1: Suppressed Grief Leading to Chronic Migraines

- **Patient:** 42-year-old woman
- **Chief Complaint:** Chronic migraines for five years, worsening during emotional distress.
- **Emotional History:** Lost her mother but never fully expressed her grief. She insisted she had "moved on" but avoided discussing her loss.

- **Observations:** Tense shoulders, clenched jaw, forced smile, teary eyes when discussing childhood.
- **Remedy: Natrum Muriaticum** – For suppressed grief and emotional withdrawal.
- **Follow-up:** After two weeks, she reported reduced headache intensity and an emotional release through dreams of her mother. Over three months, migraines significantly improved as she processed her grief.

---

**Case 2: Anger Suppression Resulting in Skin Eruptions**

- **Patient:** 28-year-old male
- **Chief Complaint:** Recurring eczema flare-ups, especially after work conflicts.
- **Emotional History:** Avoided confrontation but harboured resentment toward his boss.
- **Observations:** Clenched fists, forced politeness, jaw tightness when discussing workplace conflicts.
- **Remedy: Staphysagria** – For suppressed anger manifesting in skin conditions.
- **Follow-up:** Within a month, the eczema improved, and he started asserting himself at work. Emotional balance led to long-term skin recovery.

---

**Case 3: Performance Anxiety and Panic Attacks**

- **Patient:** 19-year-old student

- **Chief Complaint:** Severe anxiety before exams, palpitations, trembling hands.
- **Emotional History:** Fear of failure due to high parental expectations.
- **Observations:** Restless leg movement, rapid speech, sweating during consultation.
- **Remedy: Argentum Nitricum** – For anticipatory anxiety and impulsive nervous behaviours.
- **Follow-up:** After a single dose, anxiety levels dropped significantly. Over two months, he became more confident, and panic attacks ceased.

---

**Case 4: Repressed Childhood Trauma Leading to Chronic Back Pain**

- **Patient:** 50-year-old woman
- **Chief Complaint:** Chronic lower back pain with no structural abnormalities.
- **Emotional History:** History of childhood neglect and emotional suppression.
- **Observations:** Avoidance of personal history, a defensive tone when asked about family.
- **Remedy: Stramonium** – For deep-seated trauma and fear stored in the body.
- **Follow-up:** Intense emotional dreams followed by a gradual reduction in back pain over four months. She started opening up about childhood wounds.

---

**Case 5: Recurrent Tonsillitis Due to Emotional Suppression**

- **Patient:** 10-year-old boy
- **Chief Complaint:** Frequent sore throats, especially before school events.
- **Emotional History:** Shy, avoided expressing himself in class, fear of making mistakes.
- **Observations:** Soft-spoken, avoided eye contact, hesitated when asked about fears.
- **Remedy: Baryta Carbonica** – For extreme shyness and glandular affections.
- **Follow-up:** Over six months, tonsillitis frequency reduced, and he became more socially confident.

---

**Case 6: Postpartum Depression with Emotional Numbness**

- **Patient:** 32-year-old new mother
- **Chief Complaint:** Emotional detachment from her baby, extreme fatigue.
- **Emotional History:** Overwhelmed by responsibilities, felt guilty for lack of maternal emotions.
- **Observations:** Distant expression, forced smile, lack of enthusiasm while discussing motherhood.
- **Remedy: Sepia** – For post-partum emotional numbness and hormonal imbalances.
- **Follow-up:** After three weeks, she reported emotional warmth returning. Fatigue improved over two months.

---

**Case 7: Irritability and Digestive Issues Due to Work Stress**

- **Patient:** 45-year-old businessman
- **Chief Complaint:** Acid reflux, irritability, difficulty sleeping.
- **Emotional History:** High work stress, perfectionist, short-tempered.
- **Observations:** Fast speech, impatience, frequently checked his phone.
- **Remedy: Nux Vomica** – For workaholic stress, digestive disturbances, and irritability.
- **Follow-up:** Within a month, digestive issues subsided. Sleep improved as he practiced better stress management.

---

**Case 8: Fear of Abandonment Leading to Breathlessness**

- **Patient:** 26-year-old woman
- **Chief Complaint:** Sudden episodes of breathlessness, especially in relationships.
- **Emotional History:** Had experienced abandonment in childhood, developed anxiety in close relationships.
- **Observations:** Shallow breathing, frequent sighing, teary eyes while discussing relationships.
- **Remedy: Pulsatilla** – For dependency, insecurity, and emotional hypersensitivity.
- **Follow-up:** Over two months, breathlessness disappeared, and she developed healthier attachment patterns.

---

**Case 9: Suppressed Jealousy Leading to Hormonal Imbalance**

- **Patient:** 35-year-old woman
- **Chief Complaint:** Irregular periods, mood swings.
- **Emotional History:** Felt overshadowed by a sibling but never expressed it.
- **Observations:** Talkative but defensive when discussing family, avoided direct answers.
- **Remedy: Lachesis** – For suppressed jealousy and hormonal disorders.
- **Follow-up:** Within three months, menstrual cycles normalized, and emotional balance improved.

---

**Case 10: PTSD Manifesting as Chronic Nightmares**

- **Patient:** 38-year-old war veteran
- **Chief Complaint:** Nightmares, insomnia, flashbacks.
- **Emotional History:** Witnessed traumatic events but never fully processed them.
- **Observations:** Hypervigilance, sudden startle reflex, clenched jaw.
- **Remedy: Aconitum Napellus** – For acute fear, panic, and PTSD-related symptoms.
- **Follow-up:** After one month, nightmares reduced significantly. Over six months, he developed a calmer demeanour.

---

### 3. Conclusion

*These case studies illustrate how homoeopathy, combined with an understanding of emotional and psychodynamic factors, can help heal deep-rooted issues. By addressing suppressed emotions, fears, and trauma, remedies not only relieve physical symptoms but also restore emotional balance.*

---

## Chapter 27: Illness as a Failure of Adaptation: A Holistic Perspective

*Inspired by the teachings of my Guru*

In the teachings passed down by my Guru, illness is not merely a malfunction of bodily systems, nor just a biological deviation from health. Instead, it is better understood as a **failure of adaptation** — a disturbance in the subtle, dynamic equilibrium between the individual and their inner and outer environments.

When this balance breaks down — whether due to suppressed emotions, spiritual stagnation, or environmental strain — disease manifests not just in the body, but in the very field of consciousness.

---

### The Two Environments of Adaptation

The individual is not isolated, but continuously responding to two distinct environments:

---

1. The Natural Environment

*That which existed before birth*

- **Microorganisms** – Bacteria, viruses, fungi

- **Climate** – Heat, cold, humidity, wind
- **Natural Elements** – Earth, air, fire, water
- **Flora and Fauna** – Animals, plants, and ecosystem
- **Cosmic Rhythms** – Lunar cycles, planetary influences

When the individual fails to adapt to this domain — due to hereditary sensitivity, poor vitality, or suppression of natural reactions — disease arises.
For instance, a child prone to repeated colds may not just be "catching viruses" but may be expressing an internal disharmony that impairs adaptation to seasonal or microbial changes.

---

2. The Artificial Environment

*That which develops after birth*

- **Family Structures** – Parental influence, sibling dynamics
- **Relationships** – Friendships, love, intimacy, betrayal
- **Social Roles** – Expectations, careers, identity pressures
- **Cultural Norms** – Beliefs, stigmas, societal conditioning
- **Emotional Wounds** – Loss, rejection, abandonment

When the soul cannot harmonize with these forces, it experiences **emotional friction** — a tension that may eventually crystallize into physical pathology.
A patient suffering from chronic gastritis may not simply have a digestive disorder — they may be failing to metabolize emotional stress in relationships or unresolved inner conflict.

---

### The Soul: The Central Axis of Adaptation

At the heart of this model lies the **soul** — the invisible, dynamic principle that governs both mind and body. When the soul falters in its adaptive function, the mind becomes restless, and the body becomes reactive.

- **Disease** is not merely a biochemical event — it is the echo of a soul that has lost rhythm with its environment.
- **Healing** then becomes a journey of re-alignment, restoration, and return to inner harmony.

---

### Definition of Disease (From the *Organon of Medicine*)

**§11 – 6th Edition, Dr. Samuel Hahnemann:**

> *"When a person falls ill, it is only this spiritual, self-acting (automatic) vital force, everywhere present in the organism, that is primarily deranged by the dynamic influence upon it of a morbific agent inimical to life; it is only the vital force, deranged to such an abnormal state, that can furnish the organism with its disagreeable sensations and incline it to the irregular processes which we call disease."*

---

### Interpretation for Clinical and Psychodynamic Understanding

According to Hahnemann:

- **Disease is not merely a material alteration** of tissues or organs.
- It is first and foremost a **dynamic disturbance** of the **vital force** — the immaterial, life-governing energy that animates the body.

- This disturbance manifests as **discomfort (subjective symptoms)** and **irregular functioning (objective signs)**.
- The cause is **dynamic** in nature — an energetic influence, not necessarily a physical substance.

---

**Integrated View: Disease as Disturbed Harmony**

**Disease as a failure of adaptation**:

- The **vital force** is the **soul's biological expression** — the bridge between the spiritual center and the physical world.
- When this force becomes **misaligned**, the organism loses its ability to adapt.
- Symptoms are not the disease itself but are **signals of internal dissonance** — the soul crying out for realignment.

---

**Interpretation:**

Hahnemann defines disease not as a material defect but as a **dynamic disturbance** of the **vital force** — the immaterial energy that governs life. Symptoms arise only when this inner energy loses its equilibrium due to external or internal influences.

In alignment with our adaptive model, this suggests that:

- **Disease begins at the energetic level**, not the anatomical one.
- The **vital force**, when disturbed, reflects the soul's inability to maintain harmony.

- Symptoms are **not the enemy**, but a **language** through which the vital force expresses its crisis.

---

**Clinical Implications in Homoeopathy**

This understanding shifts the homoeopath's role from one who treats disease to one who **facilitates re-adaptation**. Every case becomes a story of lost harmony, and every remedy a message that gently whispers the forgotten rhythm back to the patient.

The aim of treatment, therefore, is threefold:

1. **Rebalance the individual** – Soul, mind, and body in synchrony
2. **Restore harmony with surroundings** – Natural and artificial environments
3. **Reconnect with life purpose** – The soul's unique journey

A well-selected remedy does not force the body into submission — it **resonates with the soul's pattern of disharmony** and helps the entire organism find its way back to equilibrium.

---

## Chapter (0): Shoonya: The Origin and the Return

*"Every disease has a beginning — but healing is a return.*
*A return not to the past, but to the soul, to Shoonya."*

---

**The Return to Stillness**

We began this journey in stillness — in **Shoonya** — the sacred silence before any symptom, before any suffering. Now, we arrive again at that same stillness… But this time, **transformed**.

We are not returning as the same being who began.
We return aware — having walked through the valleys of disharmony, imbalance, and pain.
We return having witnessed the **soul's signals** — first whispers in the mind, then cries in the body.

We now understand:

- That every **symptom was a messenger**
- That every **illness was an invitation**
- That **true healing** is not suppression, but **transformation**

---

**The Sacred Cycle**

Disease, as we have seen, is not merely a physical event.
It is a **failure of harmony** — a forgetting of who we truly are.

It begins when the **soul is silenced** or misaligned — by trauma, suppression, or loss of meaning.
The **mind distorts** — through fear, repression, reaction, or belief.
The **body speaks** — manifesting the inner disharmony through symptoms, illness, and syndromes.

*"The body speaks when the soul has been silenced."*

Healing, therefore, is not merely symptomatic relief.
It is the **soul's reawakening**.

The journey back from distortion to clarity, from disease to **Shoonya**.

---

### The Descent into Disease

Disease does not begin in the body.
It begins in the **disruption of soul-consciousness** — a misalignment with our deeper truth.

When the **soul forgets** its nature or is overshadowed by trauma, isolation, or suppression of being...

The **mind begins to distort** — emotions become exaggerated, thoughts reactive, identity fragmented.

Eventually, the **body bears the burden** — expressing the soul's silent scream through symptoms and syndromes.

> *"The body speaks when the soul has been silenced."*

What we call "illness" is often the **final echo** of a long-forgotten imbalance.

---

### Why End with Shoonya?

This book began in Shoonya — in the remembrance of our soul-nature.
And it must end there too, because **healing is not the destination**, but the **return** to the still point from which all balance flows.

We have walked through the psychodynamics of symptoms, through the deeper layers of pain and adaptation.
We have seen how disease begins not in the body, but in the deeper emotional and spiritual layers.

And now, we arrive again at the silence — but this time, with awareness.

Shoonya is now not just a beginning.
It is a **realization**.
We return as the **witness**, no longer fragmented, but integrated.

---

### The Pattern of Manifestation

From **Soul**, disturbance arises
→ It descends into the **Mind**, altering perceptions, beliefs, and emotions
→ It takes shape in the **Body**, where it becomes visible

This is the **sacred downward spiral of disease**.
And healing is simply the **upward return** — from physical relief, to emotional resolution, to soul realignment.

> *"True healing does not end with the disappearance of symptoms.*
> *It ends with the return to Shoonya — to the stillness from which health was first born."*

---

### Soul as the Final Healer

The physician may stimulate healing.
The remedy may guide the force.
The counselling may soothe the mind.
But **only the soul restores harmony**.

Because the soul is not ill — it is the part that **watches, waits**, and **knows**.
It is eternal. It neither decays nor reacts. It simply **is**.

Shoonya is the **soul's resting place** — the inner space where healing is complete not because the pain is gone, but because we are no longer separate from our essence.

> *"The journey through sickness was never about disease — it was about remembering who we truly are."*

---

### From the Cycle to the Center

We are no longer trapped in the cycle of cause and effect, symptom and cure.
We now rest at the center — the **zero-point** — where nothing needs to be added or removed.

In the beginning, there was Shoonya.
In the end, there is Shoonya.
And in between? A **sacred dance of forgetting and remembering**.

This is not the end.
It is the **stillness between two notes,**
the **silence between two lives,**
the **breath before the next becoming**.

> *"Health is not the absence of illness — it is the presence of soul-awareness."*

---

### Closing the Circle

Every symptom was a message.
Every remedy a tuning fork.
Every step a return toward wholeness.

From Soul → to Mind → to Body — the **descent of disharmony**
And back from Body → to Mind → to Soul — the **ascent of healing**

This is not the end.
This is the still point between cycles.
The breath between two lifetimes.
The quiet after the storm.

*"Shoonya is where the soul remembers itself.*
*And that is the beginning of everything."*

---

*"Everything begins with **Shoonya (Zero)** and ends in **Shoonya**. Health, disease, and healing are all part of this eternal cycle—emerging from the unseen, manifesting in form, and dissolving back into the infinite."*

**Special Thanks**

*I extend my heartfelt gratitude to the wonderful individuals who helped me bring The Soul of Sickness to life.*

*Publishing a first book through self-publishing is never easy, but these generous souls stood by me with selfless support and guidance:*

***Mr. Deepak Karanjikar***

***(Well Known Marathi Actor&Author of Many Books)***
***Mr. Shirish Shathe***
***Dr. Shailendra Apte***
***Mr. Bhasvan Joshi***

*Thank you for your invaluable help in making this book a reality.*

*Your belief in my vision gave this book its wings.*